PRAISE FOR MISSY CHASE LAPINE AND

Sneaky Blends

"The Sneaky Chef has done it again! In a world where we seem to have forgotten you are what you eat, *Sneaky Blends* gives us the road map to creating nutrient-dense blends that will help anyone feel more energized and be healthier."

—Michael Lewis, MD, president and founder,
Brain Health Education and Research Institute

"Say goodbye to fighting over greens and hello to healthier meals that taste incredible."

—Brooke Griffin, author of *Skinny Suppers* and founder of SkinnyMom.com

"Missy has been a champion of children's health through her innovative Sneaky Chef books—bringing easy ways to add vegetables and other nutritious foods into our kids' diets. Now with *Sneaky Blends*, we adults have a delicious chance to enjoy her signature blends and purees for ourselves! The book is beautiful to browse, and the recipes [are] so delicious, it makes healthy eating a pleasure!"

—Elizabeth Pantley, author of *The No-Cry Picky Eater Solution:
Gentle Ways to Encourage Your Child to Eat—and Eat Healthy*

"With Missy's recipes, we have no excuse for avoiding the delicious, satisfying foods we've all been neglecting. She understands flavors and texture as well as any chef and edits her recipes for a healthy experience."

—Daniel Boulud, chef/owner, The Dinex Group

"I have been immersed in the health and wellness space for fifteen years, on the fitness and the food and beverage sides. I believe that Missy's blends will trigger a nutritional revolution, by providing wonderfully tasty, nutritionally dense food products and offering superior accessible nutrition and an exceptional delivery system for all ages."

—Mark W. Wood, CEO and founder, Wolfpack Hospitality

"*Sneaky Blends* is a versatile guide that will add pizzazz to your dishes and delight your taste buds."

—Samantha Heller, registered dietitian, exercise physiologist,
and author of *The Only Cleanse*

"*Sneaky Blends* is a game changer for those of us who know how difficult it is to stay healthy when constantly on the go. Not only do these nutrient-packed purees help save precious time in the kitchen, but they also allow you to feel better about eating your favorite comfort foods."

—Phoebe Lapine, founder of FeedMePhoebe.com
and author of *The Wellness Project*

"Missy has a flair for creating healthful recipes with a boost of good-for-you nutrients. Her latest book has lots of fabulous healthy recipes that are a perfect addition to any healthy eating plan."

—Toby Amidor, MS, RD, nutrition expert
and author of *The Greek Yogurt Kitchen*

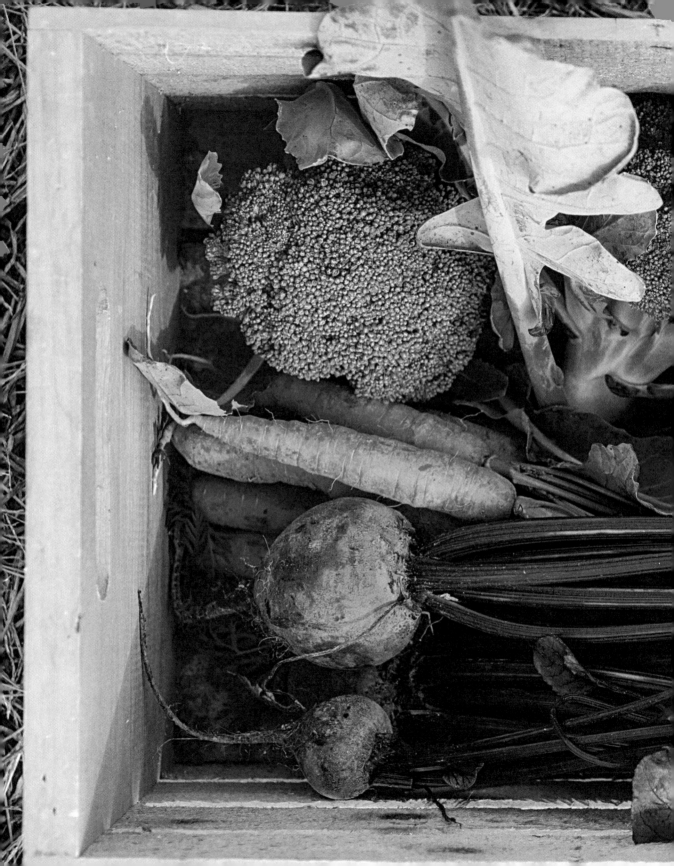

Sneaky Blends

Supercharge Your Health
with More Than 100 Recipes
Using the Power of Purees

MISSY CHASE LAPINE

PHOTOGRAPHY BY
JENNIFER MAY

NORTH STAR WAY

NEW YORK   LONDON   TORONTO   SYDNEY   NEW DELHI

North Star Way
An Imprint of Simon & Schuster, Inc.
1230 Avenue of the Americas
New York, NY 10020

First North Star Way hardcover edition September 2016

NORTH STAR WAY and colophon are trademarks of Simon & Schuster, Inc.

For information about special discounts for bulk purchases, please contact Simon & Schuster Special Sales at 1-866-506-1949 or business@simonandschuster.com

The North Star Way Speakers Bureau can bring authors to your live event. For more information or to book an event, contact the North Star Way Speakers Bureau at 1-212-698-8888 or visit our site, thenorthstarway.com.

Interior design by Jaime Putorti
Photography by Jennifer May
Food styling by Kendra McKnight
Prop styling by Raina Kattelson

Medical Disclaimer: The ideas, methods, and suggestions contained in this book are not intended to replace the advice of a nutritionist, doctor, or other trained health professional. You should consult your doctor before adopting the methods of this book. Any additions to or changes in a diet or exercise program are at the reader's discretion.

Manufactured in the United States of America

10 9 8 7 6 5 4 3 2 1

Library of Congress Cataloging-in-Publication Data

Names: Lapine, Missy Chase, author. | May, Jennifer, photographer.
Title: Sneaky blends : supercharge your health with more than 100 recipes using the power of purees / by Missy Chase Lapine ; photography by Jennifer May.
Description: New York : North Star Way, an Imprint of Simon & Schuster, Inc., [2016]
Identifiers: LCCN 2016005845| ISBN 9781501130397 (trade pbk.) | ISBN 9781501130427 (ebook)
Subjects: LCSH: Smoothies (Beverages) | Cooking (Fruit) | Cooking (Vegetables) | Blenders (Cooking) | Reducing diets. | LCGFT: Cookbooks.
Classification: LCC TX817.S636 L57 2016 | DDC 641.8/75--dc23 LC record available at http://lccn.loc.gov/2016005845

ISBN 978-1-5011-3039-7
ISBN 978-1-5011-3042-7 (ebook)

For my tireless taste testers and loves of my life,

Rick, Emily, and Sam.

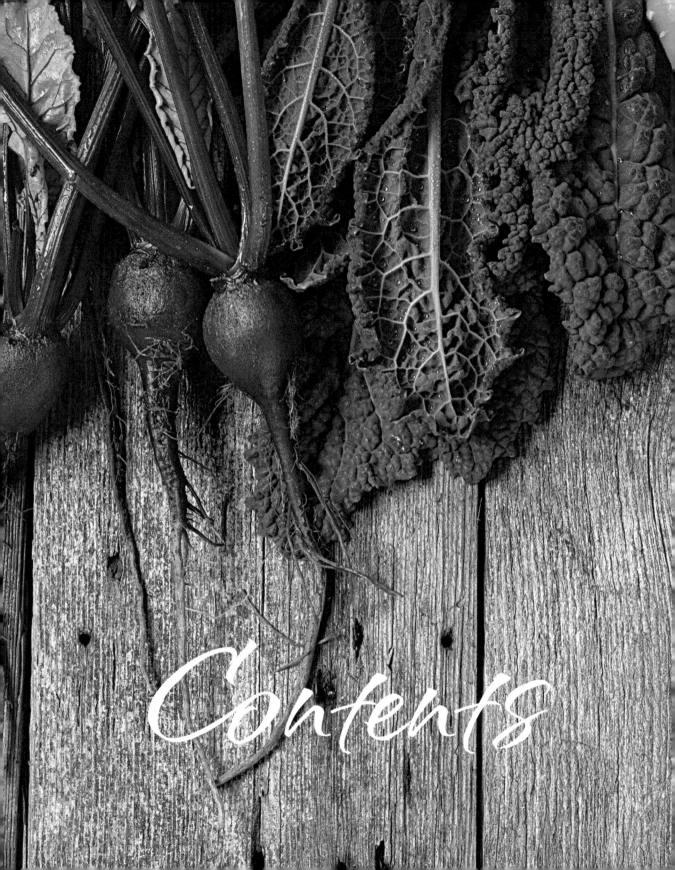

Contents

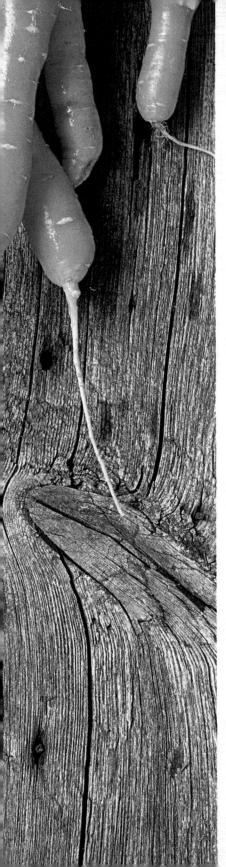

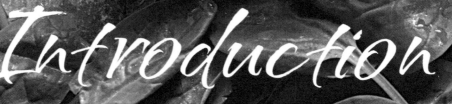

Introduction

HEALTH SNEAKS UP ON YOU

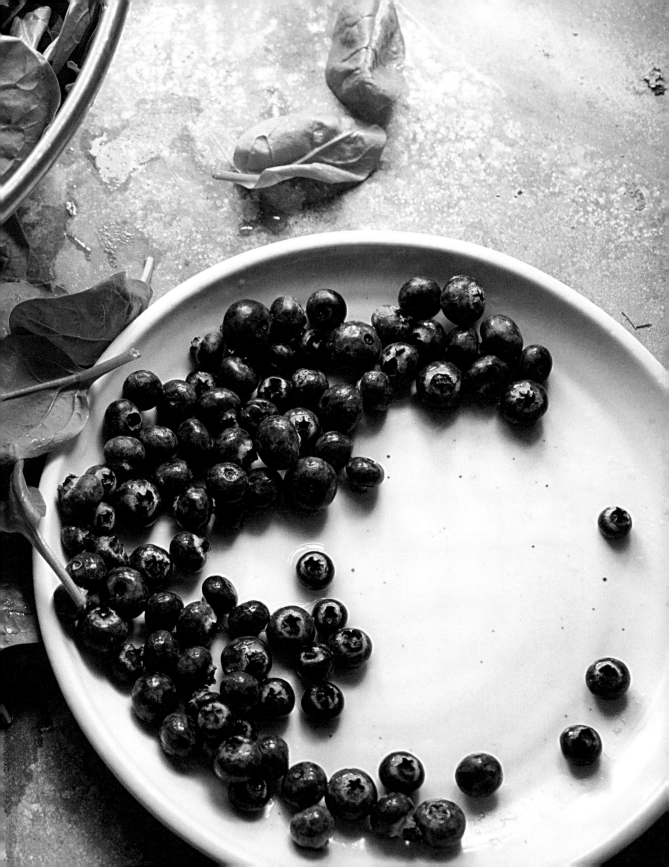

I don't know about you, but I love food too much to go through life restricting what I can eat (read: boring diet food that tastes like cardboard) just to fit into my skinny jeans. But I found a way to enjoy the decadent foods I crave, while losing weight and getting amazing nutrition. I discovered the power of blends.

Let me explain. As the author of the Sneaky Chef series, I originally created my blends as a way to pump more nutrition into my picky kids' diets, by slipping the blends into their favorite foods. But I discovered something: Moms like me all over the country were sneaking my delicious blends on themselves as a way to effortlessly get in more nutrition, feel recharged, and, get this: lose weight. As the testimonials throughout the book will tell you, it just works.

The power of blends isn't just anecdotal; research has proven they're an insanely effective tool for weight loss. A study at Pennsylvania State University found that swapping vegetable purees (aka blends) for some of the more caloric ingredients in recipes helped participants eat 357 fewer calories each day, on average—that's 2,500 calories a week. And here's the best part: Despite eating lower-calorie foods, the participants felt just as satisfied as when they ate the higher-cal, blend-free versions—and didn't detect any taste difference between the two. The blend-boosted group also "snuck" two extra servings of produce into their daily diet.

By adding blends to dishes, you also get to eat more food. (What's not to love about that?) Research published in the *American Journal of Clinical Nutrition* compared two groups of dieters—one that was told to eat a low-fat diet and another that was told to lower their overall fat intake, but also incorporate more water-rich fruits and vegetables. At the end of six months, the participants who

BLEND ('blend) *noun:* a combination of different tastes, styles, or qualities that produces an attractive or effective result.

My Sneaky Blends start with a combination of superfoods—like broccoli, peas, and spinach—that are pureed down into concentrated form (imagine the consistency of hummus). They're delicious enough to eat on their own but also are designed to be added to recipes—to make everything you eat better for you, by replacing higher-calorie ingredients with lower-calorie, antioxidant-rich blends. Think of them as condensed nutrition. They're the magical ingredient that transforms your favorite comfort foods into healthy ones.

had upped their produce intake at meals lost 33 percent more weight than the low-fat dieters, yet ate 25 percent more food. Think about it this way: Picture the sad amount of food you'd get in one of those low-fat 100-calorie packs. For the same calories, you could eat 15 cups of baby spinach. Not that you'd ever want to eat that much spinach in one sitting, but you see the point, right? The researchers noted that this type of diet is easier to stick with, too, which also helped the pounds come off.

And along with that weight loss come measurable health benefits. A University of Southern California study found that a nutrient-rich, high-veg diet not only helped participants lose a significant amount of weight over the course of one year (31 pounds, on average!), but their total cholesterol dropped by 13 points, their triglycerides fell 17 points, and their cardiac risk ratio went from 4.5 to 3.8. Their blood pressure also dropped. Weight loss in and of itself can improve all of these things, but injecting many more vitamins, minerals, and phytonutrients (health-boosting compounds found in plants) into your system in blend form increases the benefit even more.

"I actually lost the last five pounds on Missy's cleanse and people are saying how great I look. I feel so much healthier and energized—and the plan really jump-started my body and brain into craving healthy food. It was a turning point for me." —Charlotte F.

Blends are all about redefining the way you eat and live. They supercharge your health with disease-fighting antioxidants and fiber, allow you to diet without deprivation, and transform your way of eating so that the pounds you lose now—up to six in just the first three days of my plan—never return. It's a whole new, game-changing way of healthy eating.

We're all trying to eat a more plant-based diet. But you can only have so much fruit and vegetables on their own—and that's where the blends totally shine. They become a tool to get more nutrition in your foods, and replace less healthy stuff like butter, cream, and sugar—making recipes lighter. For this book, I developed fifteen different Sneaky Blends, including Carrot–Sweet Potato (see page 86), Raspberry-Beet (see page 94), Blueberry–Baby Spinach (see page 98, and Butternut Squash–Apple (see page 87), all of which are versatile and mild enough that you can use them in any sweet or savory dish.

You forget that there are beets and raspberries in your decadent chocolate cake, or that there are chickpeas in your scrumptious blueberry muffin—because everything tastes so good and is so good for you. Who can argue with that?

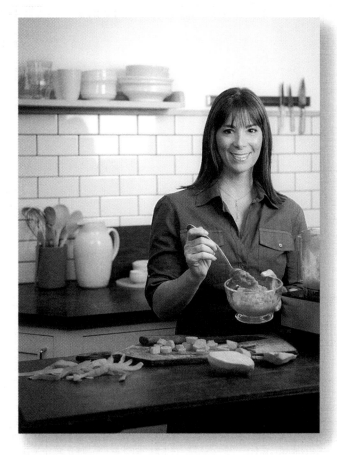

All it takes is a trip down the produce aisle and seconds of blending to make concentrated, nutrient-dense blends that make recipes invisibly lower in calories, but still incredibly satisfying. It's faster than making a salad, and easier than chopping an onion. Blends are a paradigm shift in how we think about getting our fruits and veggies, how we cook, and how we eat.

Think of these blends as next-gen juicing.

Here's more on how blends go above and beyond juicing and other big-on-promises, low-on-results diets:

✦ They don't come with a whole set of restrictions. Why slash things from your diet (carbs, protein, fiber, or actual chewable food) when you can add them in and lose weight?

"The juice cleanse I did made me irritable and shaky—and the weight I lost yo-yoed back. That didn't happen in Missy's cleanse, which was great! I had a smooth, organic energy and the blends didn't feel forced and disruptive like juicing—because they're food. They were like comfort food, actually! I lost weight, felt better, and never felt deprived." —*Hellen S.*

Look at all the fiber-rich pulp that juicing wastes—not so with my blends.

✦ They deliver satiating fiber—the kind that most juice diets throw away, leaving you with what is essentially burn-through-it-in-twenty-minutes sugar water (see image below). In fact, the glycemic load in many juices is as bad as slugging soda.

✦ You can cook with them, adding blends to everything you make. You can't do that with juices.

✦ They allow you to more than double the amount of fruit and veg you get at each meal without having to chew your way through mounds of kale and cauliflower. (Who would want to do that? Oh right, no one.) For example, 2 cups of cauliflower florets blends down to ½ cup—allowing you to pack in more servings per meal. And that's a big deal, because even though you know how many servings of produce you should be eating, the reality is this: 91 percent of Americans aren't getting enough veggies each day, and 87 percent aren't eating enough fruit, according to the Centers for Disease Control and Prevention. So even as adults, *we just don't want to eat our veggies, Mom.* Don't fool yourself about what you're getting at the chopped salad place, either: 95 percent of that bowl is lettuce, and not the powerhouse veggies you really want to have. My blends get you on a more plant-based diet, which is what every major health organization—including the National Institutes of Health and the American Heart Association—is promoting these days. They're not just a fad—they're the future.

"I was a really bad eater—I always meant to do better than I did. Missy's blends helped kick-start my healthy eating." —Michele M.

✦ They replace a third to half of the calories and fat in recipes, so you lose weight while still eating the stuff you crave. Think mac and cheese. My recipe uses Carrot–Sweet Potato Base Blend in place of much of the cheese and other unhealthy ingredients—yet it's still rich and creamy and totally hits the spot. You'll also find recipes for chicken Parm, pizza, pancakes, and decadent truffles.

✦ My blends give you a no-hype cleanse from nourishing foods that are packed with fiber and antioxidants (two of nature's best detoxers!). Antioxidants, as you may know, are substances that swoop in and neutralize free radicals—those rogue

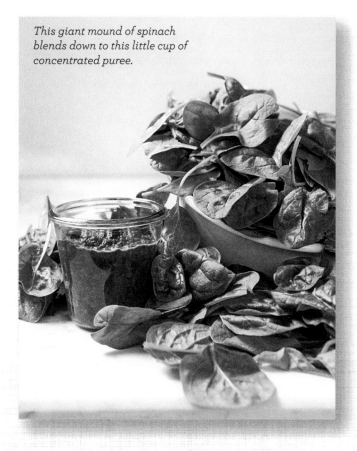

This giant mound of spinach blends down to this little cup of concentrated puree.

"Missy's 3-Day Reboot made me feel like I was getting a cleanse—but also like I was eating really well. I had good energy, didn't feel hungry, and had delicious, clean food. I actually still do it on my own two days a week because the blends are so easy to make and it keeps my weight on track." —*Elina F.*

molecules that can damage DNA and lead to a whole host of health problems. There are countless studies linking health benefits to the fruits, veggies, and legumes in my blends—yet did you know that a recent study found that no good research has been done showing that commercial juice diets actually work?

✦ They're incredibly versatile. A juice is a juice is a juice. What you see is what you get. But my Sneaky Blends can be used in multiple ways. You can add them to all sorts of recipes to bump up the nutrition and slash calories. Many blends, such as White Bean (see page 83), can also be eaten straight up all on their own, or with a few extra things added in, such as rosemary and garlic, to give them an entirely different flavor profile. You can be creative with them!

✦ Most of all, they're a way of living, eating, and cooking—not a diet. Every diet—whether we're talking about juicing or going Paleo—is a means to an end: weight loss. But once the pounds are off, then what? Sipping green juice all day is nothing like the way we eat in real life, so when you go off the plan, you're back at dietary square one. Any wonder why you always regain the weight? You're just going to fall into your old eating habits and before you know it, the numbers on the scale will start climbing again. Boosting the nutrition and weight-friendliness of the everyday foods you eat with blends is a sustainable lifestyle, not a fad diet.

HOW THIS BOOK WORKS

Ready to get blending? In Chapter 1, you'll find all the details you need to get started: items to stock up on, tips on blending and storage, and the incredible health and detoxifying benefits that the fruits, veggies, and beans in my blends have been shown to have. Then, in Chapter 2, I provide a 3-Day Reboot—a simple cleanse that uses blends as a way to get as much clean nutrition into your diet as possible, while keeping the calories low enough that you can lose up to six pounds in those three days. I find that going all-in is the best way get into the habit of using blends on an everyday basis. But if you're more interested in using them to transform your health (and recipes), you can skip the Reboot and go right to Chapter 3 (Thrive)—where I'll give you detailed advice and tools on how to easily incorporate blends into your life.

Part Two contains all the recipes you need to get blending—more than 100 of them—along with handy charts that let you know which blend is in which recipe for easy reference. Chapter 4 contains the fifteen Base Blend recipes: the basic purees that you'll add to the recipes in Chapter 5—which include your three squares plus snacks, desserts, and drinks.

Keep calm and blend on!

"This book is amazing and transformative! It merges healthy with yummy with weight loss. I can't believe how energized and happy I feel from Missy's Blends. For the first time ever, I don't feel drained trying to lose a few pounds. Nor do I feel deprived in any way. I am really enjoying food and life at a whole new level!" —Brigitte M.

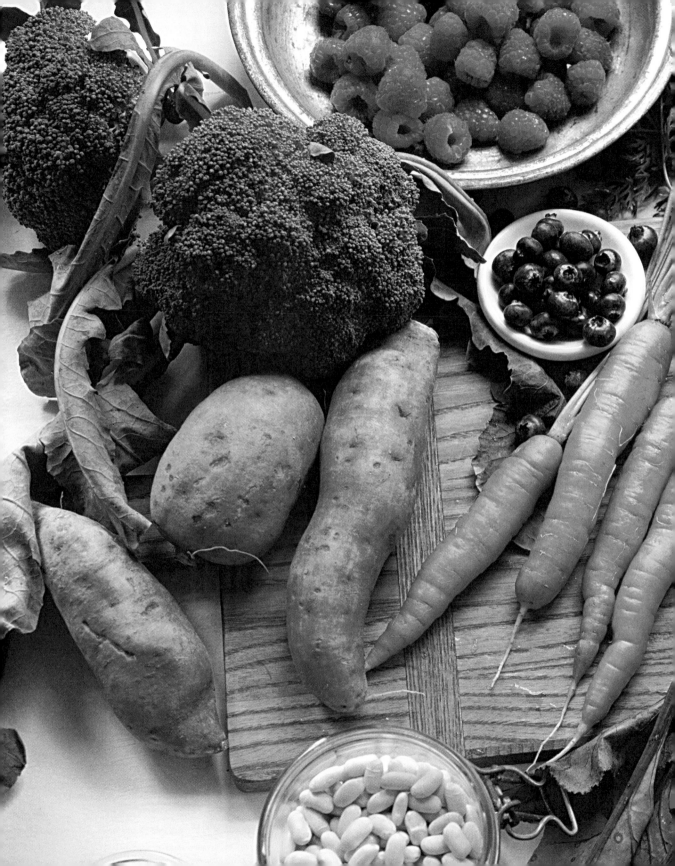

Part 1:
The Plan

Welcome to the most satisfying—and sneakily nutritious—*un*diet around. This part of the book has all the tips and tools you need to get started, plus a Reboot plan to jump-start weight loss and detailed information on how to incorporate blends into not just the recipes in this book but your own favorite dishes, from soups to pastas to brownies.

Chapter 1:
Prep

EVERYTHING YOU NEED
TO START BLENDING

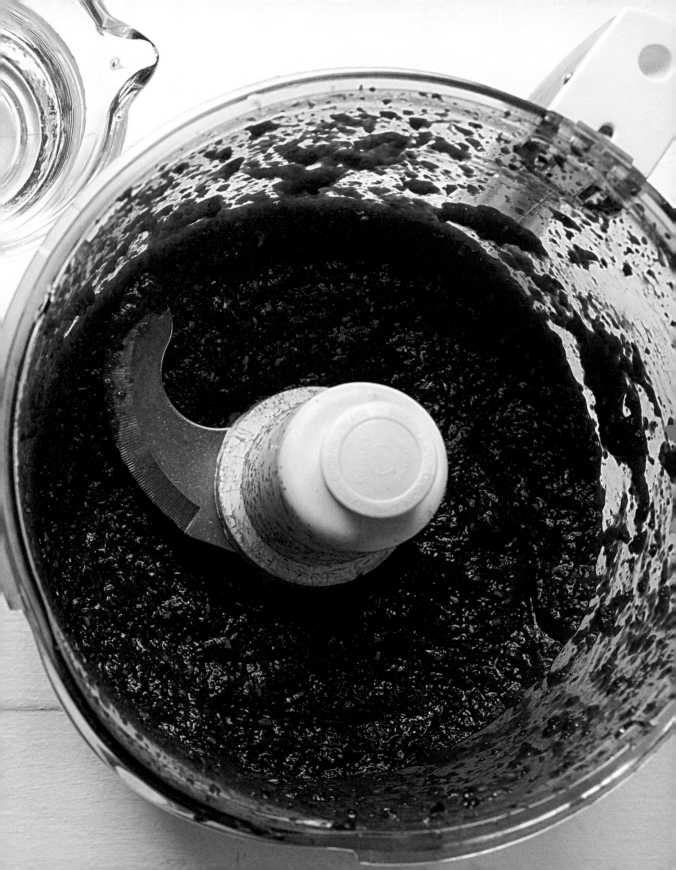

Making a blend is faster and easier than making a salad or even extracting a juice. Most of my signature recipes take just minutes to prepare and require minimal equipment, ingredients, and cleanup. But there are some essential kitchen items you'll need to have on hand for making them an everyday part of your life.

The lists and tips you'll find in this chapter will set you up with all the basics. Again, there is nothing fancy you need to own; you probably already have most of the equipment in your kitchen. But being prepared is a key part of success on this—or any—healthy-eating plan. So: Let's do a little shopping and gathering.

EQUIPMENT YOU'LL NEED

✦ *High-powered blender or food processor with a capacity of at least 3 cups* Standard blenders require far too much liquid to mix up your blends properly, so a high-powered one is best—and you don't need to shell out $400 on a super-fancy one. There are plenty of affordable options out there. Look for a blender with a plunger, which is important for pushing produce down so it blends well. You can also use a food processor, but you may need to add a bit more water to get things moving, and the blend won't be quite as smooth as those made in a high-powered blender. It will still do the trick, though. I made the recipes for all my books with the same $39 gadget.

✦ *Rubber-tipped spatula* To scoop out the blends—you don't want to waste a drop.

✦ *Large soup pot with a lid* A few of the blend recipes require a quick steam before you blitz the veggies.

✦ *Ceramic nonstick skillet* Regular nonstick cookware contains chemicals that release when heated. So do your body a favor and invest in a ceramic-coated pan such as Cerastone™ or Cerapan™ brand, which doesn't contain any of these potentially harmful chemicals.

✦ *Fine-mesh stainless-steel strainer* (Not a colander.) Several of the recipes in this book call for straining liquid, so this kitchen tool will come in handy.

✦ *Steamer basket* It's an inexpensive item that's worth buying if you don't have one, because steaming produce in a basket allows you to retain much more of the nutrients than boiling them directly in water does.

✦ *Storage containers* To stash your blends in so you'll have them ready to go for snacks or recipes. Be sure to buy containers that are BPA and phthalate free.

✦ *Measuring cups and spoons* Sure, you'll need them for prepping recipes, but I also recommend using them for portioning out servings, so your calories stay in line.

✦ *Vegetable peeler* You'll need it for peeling veggies like zucchini and squash.

✦ *Mini muffin tin* Some of the sweets call for this cute little guy—and believe me, you're gonna want to make them. (Cough, donuts, cough.)

✦ *Covered ice cube trays for storing extra blends in the freezer* They give you a convenient premeasured amount. (Two cubes equal about ¼ cup of blend.) And yes, all of the blends freeze brilliantly!

✦ *Sandwich-size resealable plastic bags* Use them as an alternative to ice cube trays—or for freezing larger amounts of blends at once. Be sure to label and date them, and jot down the amount of blend in each baggie. I recommend freezing in ¼-cup portions, which will thaw quickly and match up with the amounts called for in many of the recipes.

✦ *Portable coffee cups with lids*—like the kind you get your Starbucks in. You can pick them up at a restaurant supply store or on Amazon. Or, if you'd rather, you can purchase reusable ones. They're great for the 3-Day Reboot, when you're just having doctored-up versions of straight blends. You can carry all your meals and snacks around with you—without looking silly—and most are microwavable.

✦ *Spiralizer* These gadgets are very popular. You use it to make spaghetti-like noodles out of zucchini and other veggies. And while, yes, it is a specialty item, you can pick one up for about $10 and make a plate full of yummy, faux pasta that has more phytonutrients than actual noodles and a fraction of the calories. My recipe for Zucchini Pasta Piccata on page 158 calls for this—and trust me, you'll get loads of use out of it for other dishes. But in a pinch, you can use a vegetable peeler to get a more fettuccine-like look.

STOCK UP

Here's a shopping list for the blends you'll be making throughout the plan. I'm only including foods that keep pretty well and that you'll be using all the time—so you can go ahead and stock up on them now. You'll notice that some

TRY THIS!

Leave your blender or food processor out on the kitchen counter all the time. If it's there, it's guaranteed you'll use it—as opposed to having to lug that big old appliance you got for your wedding out of a closet. In sight, in mind.

of the items appear on multiple lists. I did that by design to allow you to buy that item in whatever form (fresh or frozen) you prefer. (I'll give you a more specific list of items for the 3-Day Reboot, which will include everything—fresh or otherwise—that you'll need for those few days.)

FRESH PRODUCE

Apples	Broccoli	Lemons
Avocado	Butternut squash	Limes
Baby spinach	Carrots	Raspberries
Baby kale	Cauliflower	Sweet onions
Beets	Cucumber	Sweet potatoes
Blueberries	Garlic	Zucchini

FRIDGE

Ground flaxseed	Unsweetened	Organic omega-3
Plain, low-fat Greek	plant-based milk,	eggs
yogurt	such as almond	Parmesan cheese
	or coconut	(not pre-grated)
	(carrageenan free)	

TRY THIS! Don't just buy any old Parmesan cheese—look for wedges labeled Parmigiano-Reggiano that also have the letters D.O.P. on the rind, which means it's the real imported Italian deal. It's pricier than regular Parm, but it's *so* much more flavorful that it's totally worth it—and you won't need to use as much, which is good for your wallet and your waist.

TRY THIS! Look for baking soda that's labeled "aluminum free." It's widely available and eliminates that slightly off, tinny taste in baked goods. Plus, who wants to eat aluminum?

FREEZER FRUITS AND VEG

Broccoli florets

Blueberries

Butternut squash

Cauliflower florets

Mixed berries

Raspberries

Sweet peas

Sweet potatoes

PANTRY

Almond butter

Black peppercorns

Boxed whole, peeled
  tomatoes in juice
  (BPA-free)

Brown rice

Chia seeds (black or
  white)

Canned 100% pure
  pumpkin (not pie
  mix)

Canned beets (BPA-
  free)

Canned black beans
  (BPA-free) or
  dried black beans

Canned chickpeas
  (BPA-free) or
  dried chickpeas

Canned white beans
  (BPA-free) or
  dried white beans

Cocoa nibs

Cocoa powder
  (unsweetened,
  non–Dutch
  processed)

Dried oregano

Extra-virgin olive
  oil

Ground Ceylon
  cinnamon

Low-sodium chicken
  or vegetable broth
  (BPA-free and
  MSG-free)

Nonstick cooking
  spray

Peanut butter,
  all natural (or
  Sneaky Chef
  No-Nut Butter*)

Protein powder
  (unsweetened
  plain or vanilla)

Pure maple syrup

Pure vanilla extract

Raw honey

Raw pistachios

Rolled oats

Sea salt

White whole wheat
  flour or whole
  grain *pastry* flour

Whole grain pasta
  (whole wheat or
  gluten free)

* This is my peanut butter alternative, for those with nut allergies. It's made with roasted golden peas. You can buy it at thesneakychef.com.

TRY THIS! Wondering what the heck raw honey is? It's unpasteurized and unfiltered—which means it's less processed than traditional honey, and may have more health benefits, too. The heat used during the pasteurization process reduces honey's natural antifungal and antioxidant properties. But because raw honey doesn't get heated (or isn't exposed to heat that high), you get more of its immune-boosting, disease-fighting action. Just don't give to babies under one year old.

TRY THIS! Tomatoes packaged in boxes—also called Tetra Paks—are a better way to go than canned. Why? Because canned tomatoes have one of the highest levels of BPA of any canned food. The acidity in the tomatoes actually leaches this chemical from the can. Glass jars are another good option.

MY FROZEN FOOD MANIFESTO

When it comes to buying produce, people always ask me: "What's better, fresh fruits and veggies or frozen?" My answer is that unless you're able to get local produce in season (and ideally organic) I prefer going frozen most of the time. And I'll tell you why:

✦ Frozen fruits and veggies are often *fresher* than the fresh stuff. That's because they're picked and flash frozen at their absolute prime. Who knows how long that zucchini and cauliflower have been languishing in the produce section—and in transit before that?

✦ They're less time-consuming. Can you imagine shelling your own peas? Good luck with that. Frozen veggies have also been blanched, which saves you the step of having to steam them.

✦ They're cheaper. Trust me, I've done the math!

✦ They're easier to blend, because they've been partially cooked already.

✦ They're available all year-round.

✦ There's an incredible variety of them! These days, you can find everything from sweet potatoes to frozen cauliflower.

✦ They won't spoil nearly as fast as the stuff in your veggie crisper.

So load up! Frozen is where it's at.

Two veggies I *do* recommend buying fresh are baby spinach and baby kale. They have a milder flavor than the frozen kind and aren't nearly as dense. And it's so easy and inexpensive to grab a bag of prewashed greens.

WHEN TO GO ORGANIC

If you can swing it, I recommend buying organic produce to avoid pesticides. But I get that it may not be realistic to purchase 100 percent of your fruits and veg this way—so here's a list of foods to prioritize. They're best to get organic because their conventional counterparts contain the highest amounts of pesticides. They used to be called the "dirty dozen," but the list was recently updated by the Environmental Working Group (a nonprofit environmental research organization) to add a few more polluted foods. The EWG estimates that you can reduce your pesticide intake by as much as 80 percent if you steer clear of the top offenders. I've also included a rundown of the fruits and veggies that tend to be lowest in pesticides. Don't feel compelled to buy them organic.

Best foods to buy organic

1. Strawberries
2. Apples
3. Nectarines
4. Peaches
5. Celery
6. Grapes
7. Cherries
8. Spinach
9. Tomatoes
10. Sweet bell peppers
11. Cherry Tomatoes
12. Cucumbers
13. Hot peppers
14. Kale

Foods with the lowest pesticide levels

1. Avocados
2. Sweet corn
3. Pineapples
4. Cabbage
5. Sweet peas (frozen)
6. Onions
7. Asparagus
8. Mangos
9. Papayas
10. Kiwi
11. Eggplant
12. Honeydew melon
13. Grapefruit
14. Cantaloupe
15. Cauliflower

I don't know about you, but I have a hard time memorizing this whole long list. My go-to rule that I actually *can* remember: Generally, fruits and veggies with tough skins are the safer ones because the skins protect the inner flesh from chemicals.

TRY THIS! Look for non-GMO canola oil and corn and soy products— like tofu and soy milk. These three foods are said to be highest in genetically modified organisms (GMOs), which may have negative health effects.

BLEND PREP POINTERS

Some blends come together literally in thirty seconds, and others take around fifteen to twenty minutes, if you're using fresh veggies that you need to pre-steam. And as a master blender (I've been developing blends and recipes that use them for ten years), I have some tried-and-true advice that can help you put them together better and faster.

✦ Steam fresh produce, rather than boiling it in water. You'll retain nutrients that would otherwise leach into the water and just get tossed.

✦ If you're using frozen vegetables, you can skip the steaming part altogether—because they've already been precooked a little. Simply pour hot water over them and throw them into your blender.

✦ Label and date all your blends. They keep in the fridge for three days and will last for up to three months in the freezer.

✦ Freeze extras in ¼-cup sizes. Smaller amounts thaw faster—and because most of the recipes call for ¼ to ½ cup of blend, you'll have pre-measured portions at the ready. If you freeze in ice cube trays, two cubes are the equivalent of ¼ cup.

✦ Keep in mind that frozen blends work best in recipes where they're used as an ingredient—as opposed to being something you eat more straight up, which are better when fresh.

TRY THIS! I like to use low-fat Greek yogurt, rather than nonfat, because it doesn't have quite as many calories as the full-fat kind, but still contains some of the beneficial fatty acids that have been skimmed off the 0% variety—fatty acids that have been linked to weight loss and smaller waist circumference.

THE SUPERFOODS INSIDE YOUR BLENDS

I picked the ingredients in my signature Base Blends because they're versatile and can be used in lots of different recipes. They're also easy to find in any grocery store and are incredibly satiating—a must for any healthy eating plan. But above all, they are nutritional superstars. Take a look at some of the benefits you'll reap from these good guys.

Beets They're popping up on menus everywhere—and their health benefits are incredible. Beets contain a group of phytochemicals called betalains, which have powerful antioxidant, as well as anti-inflammatory and liver-detoxifying abilities. They also boost cell repair and regeneration. And the high fiber content of beets improves digestion and regularity, expediting the elimination of toxins. There's even some evidence that the compounds in beets may improve blood flow, energy, and athletic performance. If you're not a beet lover, their flavor is not front and center in my blends—so don't pass them by. I've converted so many people!

Black Beans Recent research has linked this legume with improved digestion and gut health by helping to feed the "good bugs" in your system. There's also strong evidence that black beans can help with weight loss, thanks to their high fiber and protein content—a unique combo that makes them particularly satisfying. In fact, one cup of black beans packs half of your recommended daily fiber intake—and a third of your protein requirement. They've also been shown to lower the risk of diabetes, heart disease, and colon cancer. Black beans are superstar sources of iron, folate, vitamin B, and omega-3 fatty acids, as well.

"Making the Blends is so easy. All you need are a couple of ingredients—and I love that they're 100 percent real, whole food. There are so many juice diets and cleanses where you don't know what's in there—or what isn't in there. I can make a big batch of several blends all at once and freeze extras. Super fast." —Sue A.

Blueberries Blueberries are among the fruits highest in antioxidants, according to a USDA study. Also, research has found that freezing blueberries (which my recipes call for) doesn't affect their antioxidant levels. In fact, a South Dakota State University study actually found that frozen blueberries may have a higher, more bioavailable concentration of anthocyanins (a group of antioxidant compounds) than fresh ones. They're also one of the most nutrient-dense fruits—loaded with vitamins A and C, zinc, potassium, iron, calcium, magnesium, and fiber—and have even been shown to help reduce belly fat.

Broccoli This green guy is loaded with detoxing glucosinolates, a group of phytonutrients that help obliterate and remove harmful contaminants from your body. And while some forms of cooking can destroy these beneficial compounds, steaming has been found to be the best at retaining them—which is part of the reason I recommend prepping broccoli this way, as opposed to boiling or blanching. Broc is also very high in protein, fiber, and calcium—and just half a cup delivers 100 percent of the recommended daily value of vitamin C, an antioxidant that boosts immunity, lowers heart disease risk, and may prevent cancer. Overall, it's one of the most nutrient-rich foods we can eat.

Butternut Squash Did you know that butternut squash is a rich source of omega-3s? It's true. And even though it's a starchy vegetable, about half of those starches are a type that research has shown to have strong antioxidant and anti-inflammatory powers. They may also help regulate insulin levels. Butternut squash is rich in vitamins A and C, energizing B vitamins, as well as fiber.

Cauliflower The phytonutrients in this cruciferous vegetable help reduce oxidative stress and lower inflammation in the body—both of which support your body's natural detox process. It's also loaded with folate, fiber, and vitamin C—which some research has shown can promote fat loss. I also love cauliflower because it adds a lot of bulk but has so few calories. An entire medium-size head of this veggie only has 147 calories.

Carrots Those rabbits are on to something! Not only do carrots boast high amounts of carotenoids—antioxidants that promote eye health and protect against certain cancers—they also contain glutathiones, compounds that bind to toxins and help clear them from your body. (They're known for their liver-detoxifying powers.) Plus, carrots are rich in polyacetylenes, phytonutrients that work in tandem with carotenoids to prevent oxidative damage and reduce cancer risk. And can we talk about their gorgeous hue? Research shows that orange/yellow produce is the most protective against heart disease compared to other color groups of fruit and veg (like red and purple). A study published in the *British Journal of Nutrition* found that *just 2 baby carrots* (25 grams) contain enough of this good-for-you phytonutrient to reduce the risk of heart disease by 32 percent—and the more you eat, the farther your odds drop.

Chickpeas These legumes are inexpensive, incredibly nutritious, and deeply satisfying. Studies have consistently linked chickpea consumption (or eating any legume, for that matter) to reduced body mass index (BMI) because they contain slow-digesting carbs and lots of fiber and protein and are lower in energy density, all of which support weight control and weight loss. Additionally, about two thirds of the fiber in chickpeas is the insoluble type that soaks up unwanted toxins in your digestive tract and helps ferry them out of your system. They're also an amazing source of folate, tryptophan, magnesium, and iron, which crank up energy levels, boost brainpower, and guard against heart disease and cancer.

Kale I've been blending kale since long before it became the darling of the produce aisle. It's an excellent source of a group of phytonutrients called gluco-sinolates. When glucosinolates are digested, your body converts them into a compound that is particularly effective at eradicating chemicals and toxins in the foods you eat and drink—by acting directly on your genes. Kale glucosinolates have also been shown to have a host of powerful "anti" properties: They are antiviral, anti-infective, anti-inflammatory, and anticarcinogenic, to name a few. Hype well deserved, if you ask me.

Peas Green peas are surprisingly satiating. In fact, one cup of them contains more protein than a large egg. They're also a good source of fiber, vitamins C and K, potassium, and iron—nutrients that support immunity, fight colds, protect against heart disease and all types of cancer, strengthen bones, and rev up your energy level. And they're high in omega-3 fatty acids.

Pumpkin Like other orange-colored produce, such as carrots and sweet potatoes, pumpkin is rich in beta-carotene, an antioxidant that helps neutralize free radicals and has been linked to cancer prevention. I often use 100 percent pure canned pumpkin, rather than go through the hassle of chopping and roasting fresh pumpkin. There's good evidence that the canned stuff is just as nutritious as—if not more than—fresh. So why not save yourself the time? Just be sure not to get the sweetened pie filling kind.

Raspberries Raspberries are a potent source of ellagic acid, a flavonoid that binds to carcinogens and neutralizes them. (It's actually used medicinally as a cancer fighter.) Ellagic acid also has an anti-inflammatory effect that may impact fatty tissues in the body, thereby lowering the risk of obesity.

Spinach Spinach is a nutrient powerhouse. It contains twice as much iron as most other greens and is an excellent source of calcium, folic acid, and vitamins A and C. It also has a high beta-carotene content, which most people think only comes from orange vegetables. This offers great protection against asthma, all kinds of cancer, and heart disease. Additionally, spinach contains

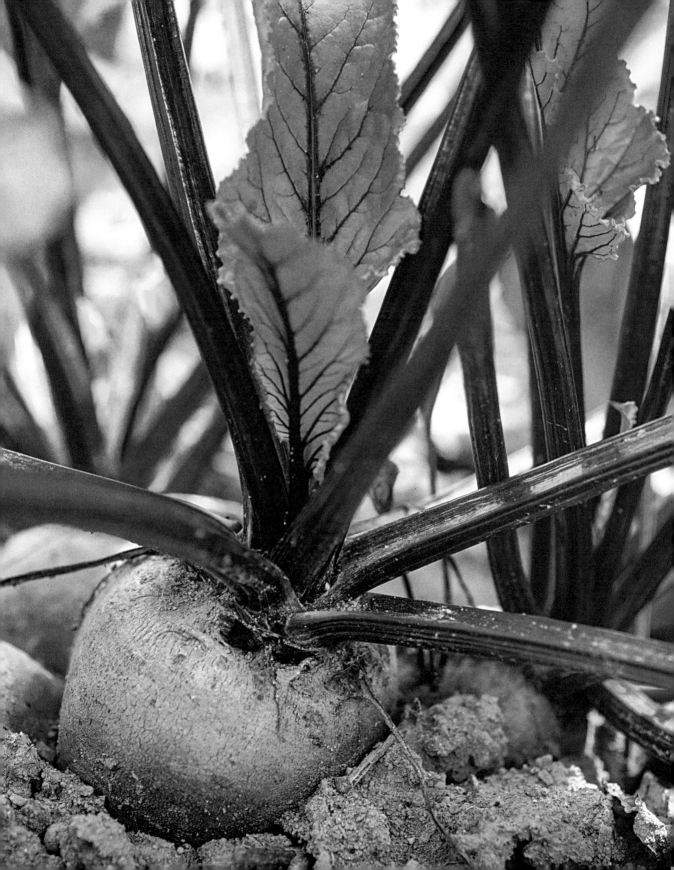

newly discovered compounds called glycoglycerolipids. Their purpose is to help the photosynthesis process; but research has also found that the glyco-glycerolipids from spinach can actually protect the lining of the digestive tract from damage, particularly damage caused by inflammation.

Sweet Potatoes For starters, they're way more weight friendly than regular spuds—one cup of white potatoes causes a blood sugar spike-and-crash (leading to increased hunger and overeating) similar to eating a handful of jelly beans! The higher fiber content in sweet potatoes blunts this effect, while still delivering the filling, satisfying comfort food you crave. That's why they're often called the "anti-diabetic" food, because they actually *stabilize* blood sugar levels. Sweet potatoes are also loaded with beta-carotene, fiber, B vitamins, calcium, potassium, and iron. And get this: Research has shown that when the cyanidins, peonidins, and other phytonutrients in sweet potatoes pass through your digestive tract, they may lower the possible health risk from toxins like heavy metals (such as lead and mercury that may sneak into your diet) and oxygen radicals.

White Beans This is a catchall term that includes navy, butter, and cannellini beans. As with black beans, they're incredibly satisfying, nutritious, and inexpensive; and they have been shown to support weight loss, thanks to their one-two punch of protein and fiber. White beans are also a good source of molybdenum, a trace element that your body needs to make and activate many of its natural detoxifying enzymes. And research shows they may lower your risk of heart disease and cancer. I also use them in my blends because their consistency adds an amazing creaminess to dishes—without adding cream.

Zucchini In terms of calories, they're a dieter's dream. One large zucchini has just 55 calories. Blending them allows you to add tons of bulk to your meal while adding very few calories. They're also high in fiber, manganese, vitamin

C, and potassium, and they have been found to protect against diseases such as asthma, certain cancers, high blood pressure, and heart disease. Some evidence even suggests they can jack up energy levels, help you think more clearly, and promote a happier disposition.

MORE POWERHOUSE FOODS YOU'LL FIND IN MY RECIPES

While they're not part of my Base Blends, I lean heavily on these super-good-for-you items in the meals, snacks, and treats you'll be eating.

Chia Seeds Tiny, but mighty! Chia seeds are loaded with system-cleansing fiber: 1 tablespoon delivers 5 grams of it, or about 20 percent of your daily requirement, as well as omega-3 fatty acids that gobble up free radicals and guard against cell damage. They also expand in your system, which may sound a little scary but really just means that they'll keep you feeling fuller, longer. Result: You'll eat less and lose weight faster.

Cinnamon This spice has been used for both culinary and medicinal purposes since 2800 B.C. And even small amounts of Ceylon cinnamon (as opposed to the cassia type that's sold as generic cinnamon in many stores) have been shown to have strong antioxidant and free-radical-scavenging properties. It may also help lower blood glucose levels, blood pressure, and cholesterol.

Cocoa The polyphenols (a group of phytochemicals) in cocoa are extremely potent—more potent than those found in green tea and red wine. They help increase the amount of good gut bacteria in the digestive tract and have anti-inflammatory powers that may lower the risk of a host of diseases, including heart disease, cancer, and metabolic disorders. Of course, I'm talking about the kind of cocoa you'd find in unsweetened cocoa powder or high-quality dark chocolate—not a Kit Kat.

Flaxseed Dubbed "one of the most powerful plant foods on the planet," flaxseed is loaded with both soluble and insoluble fiber and healthy omega-3 fats and is the richest source of lignans, a class of antioxidant that's been shown to reduce the odds of cardiovascular disease, diabetes, cancers, arthritis, autoimmune diseases, and neurological problems. There's also strong evidence that it can make your scale numbers drop. One study found that the "good" fat and fiber in 3 to 4 tablespoons of flaxseed helped dieters lose 37 percent more weight—including a significant amount of belly fat—compared to those who didn't do flax.

Strawberries These juicy red guys contain an astonishing array of phytonutrients. In fact, in a ranking of fruits and veggies by the Centers for Disease Control and Prevention, strawberries came in as the fourth most nutrient-dense fruit. Research suggests that they activate a protein called Nrf2 that increases antioxidant levels inside your cells and removes toxins. That helps explain the bevy of evidence that strawberry consumption helps reduce inflammation, heart disease, and cancer risk and boost brain health.

TRY THIS! Keep raw nuts in the freezer. You can use them directly from the freezer—no need to thaw—and they'll keep much longer than they will in the pantry. I also find that when you eat them as a snack this way, you eat them more slowly.

WHAT IS DETOXING, ANYWAY?

Detox is a huge buzzword right now—and everyone is all excited about the idea of cleansing their system. But few people know what it really means. I've done a lot of digging into this subject, but I thought it better to have a medical expert give you a quick primer to explain how detox works and how blends in particular can help. Here's the straight scoop from Pamela Peeke, M.D., an assistant clinical professor of medicine at the University of Maryland School of Medicine and author of *The Hunger Fix: The Three-Stage Detox and Recovery Plan for Overeating and Food Addiction.*

The first thing you should know is that your body actually does a masterful job detoxing itself, thank you very much—through your liver, kidneys, G.I. tract, and even your skin. They help neutralize and eliminate chemicals and other potentially harmful substances. If someone blows cigarette smoke in your face, for example, your body immediately starts working to rid itself of those toxins. In fact, you have a whole internal scanning system that's continually on the lookout for viruses and chemicals and anything bad. But you can definitely help the process along through your diet, by getting plenty of these two things:

Fiber. Fiber is like Uber—it picks up toxins in your system and drives them out of your body. It also helps things move through your system faster, which limits the amount of time that chemicals like BPA, mercury and pesticides stay in your body. The more quickly they go through you, the less chance they have to cause harm. Fiber is also terribly important for your microbiome—the ecosystem of bacteria that live in your G.I. tract and have a huge impact on your weight and health. You've got about 100 trillion bacteria in your gut and that flora must be kept in a specific balance. When we eat crap—and not just sugar, salt, and fat, but also preservatives and chemicals—it causes inflammation in the lining of our gut that then spreads throughout the body, like a domino effect. Inflammation, as you may know, is the root cause of almost every disease. The so-called good bugs in your microbiome love fiber, particularly insoluble fiber—the kind that passes through your stomach without being broken down. They feed off of it and keep the population of healthy bacteria down there strong. Those good bugs, in turn, produce short-chain fatty acids that reduce inflammation—and the irritating toxins that cause it. And there are specific foods—many of which are in this book—that contain the type of fiber your microbiota love, such as bananas, beans, sweet potatoes, yams, squash, beets, and carrots.

Phytonutrient-rich foods. They help facilitate the process by which your body takes a toxin and neutralizes it, so it can safely be excreted. It's a three-phase process that happens in your liver—which does most of the heavy lifting when it comes to detoxifying everything from alcohol and medications to air pollution and pesticides. Phytonutrients in the healthy fruits, veggies, and other foods you eat decrease the carcinogenicity and mutagenicity (changes to your DNA) of toxins and bind to them, making them ready to finally get out of your system. Broccoli, cauliflower, carrots, kale, berries, beans, sweet potato, and other foods you'll find in the blends all facilitate this part of the process. They can also help repair any DNA damage that's been caused. Finally, transporters that are present in almost every part of your body move those detoxified substances in and out of cells and through your body to your kidneys and colon, where they ultimately meet their, well, *end.*

TRY THIS! You know what else fiber does for you, aside from keeping you satisfied and helping to cleanse your system? It may also reduce the net effect of carbohydrates in your food, thereby reducing their glycemic load.

LET'S TALK NEXT STEPS

Now that you're all stocked up and ready to fire up your blender—and drop some serious weight—turn the page and get started on my 3-Day Reboot. Again, if your goal is simply to inject more nutrition into your everyday food, skip right to page 78 and begin making your blends—and the meals, snacks, and desserts that use them.

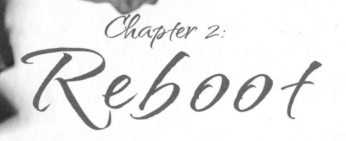

Chapter 2:

Reboot

DETOX WITHOUT DEPRIVATION—
AND LOSE UP TO 6 POUNDS
IN 3 DAYS WITH
MY BLENDS CLEANSE™

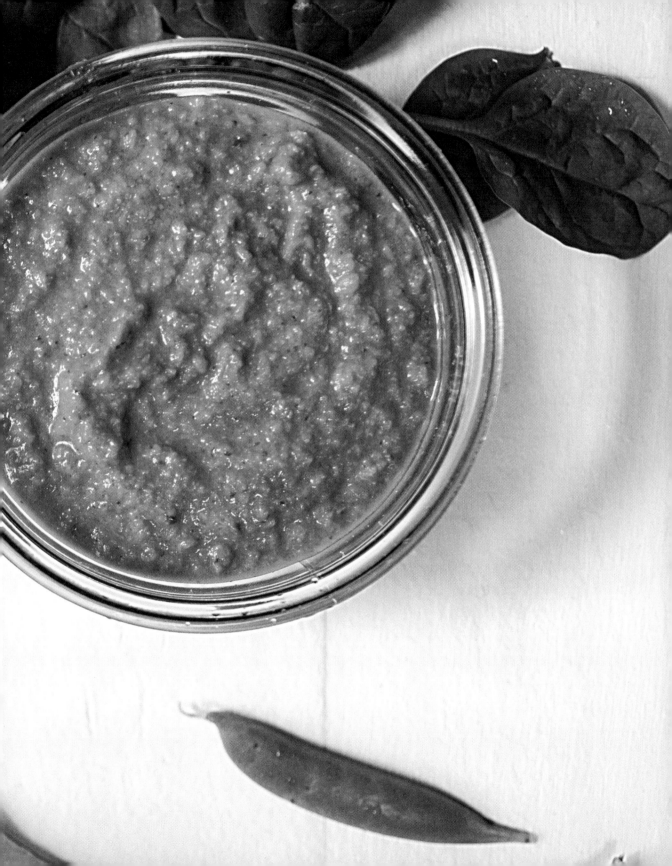

Sometimes in life we just need a do over—and this is yours. For the next seventy-two hours, you're going to cut out all the crap so many Americans put into their bodies every day—namely processed foods that are high in sugar, salt, unhealthy fats, and chemicals—and eat only blends made from whole foods. Delicious blends, I should add! Seriously: One woman who did the Reboot liked the Maple–Sweet Potato Cleanse Blend (page 45) so much she served it as a Thanksgiving side dish, and it disappeared faster than any other dish she served. In the process, you'll lose up to six pounds—and possibly even more if you have a lot of weight to drop, or are a guy. (It tends to fall away much more quickly than on someone who only has five pounds to lose.)

"I've done a lot of cleanses and this is the only one where I didn't think, 'Thank god it's over!' at the end. It's hard to diet when you're starving. You go crazy and cheat. And that's the biggest pro of this plan. Missy's blends are so physically and mentally satiating—you feel like you're eating real meals, because you are—which made the plan easier to stick with. I lost several pounds in just three days." —Eric S.

I've found that this Blends Cleanse™ phase really helps people go all in: It's an immersion into the world of blends. You get into the habit of prepping Base Blends and eating super-clean, phytonutrient-dense produce. I developed the Reboot after getting sick on a juice cleanse. I felt run-down and foggy and had terrible migraines. I wanted an alternative way to give my body a rest from the heavy, not-so-healthy foods I'd been eating; yet I found that trying to crunch my way through tons of whole fruits and vegetables was rough on my system. So rather than adding small amounts of my blends to recipes, I tried eating them almost as is—and it was a revelation.

Unlike most juice cleanses, this plan will not leave you feeling exhausted, cranky, and ravenous. Just the opposite, actually. I developed each of the recipes to be not just low-cal, but also high in fiber and protein—as well as providing megadoses of antioxidants, which help your body detoxify itself. (See page 23 for more on that.) Bonus: Every dish in the Reboot phase is gluten free and vegetarian.

Blitzing your blends also makes those amazing phytonutrients more bioavailable—because more of the cell walls have been broken down—and gives your digestive system a bit of a break, too. Yet unlike juice diets, blends are truly satiating because in addition to the fiber they contain, they're more "chewable," which slows down the eating process that research shows can help you eat less. It also triggers the release of digestive chemicals that ultimately send the "I'm full!" message to your brain. A study in the *American Journal of Clinical Nutrition* found that participants who took the time to really chew their food ate 12 percent less than those who did not—and they had higher levels of the gut hormones that help control appetite. Slurp your meal through a straw in five seconds and how likely do you think you are to feel

"I just turned forty and was having a problem keeping a bit of extra weight off. I lost those four pounds in just a few days and really feel the difference of cutting out the processed foods I had in my life. I've never done a cleanse before, because the idea just didn't seem appealing, but I didn't feel deprived at all!" —Nicole G.

satisfied? Not very. With blends, you also don't have to expend as much energy digesting your food, which makes it easier on your gastrointestinal tract than eating the same foods in whole form.

If you can, take a few days before you do the 3-Day Reboot to cut back on artificial sweeteners, sugar, salt, fatty foods like meat and cheese, alcohol, and processed foods. And if you're a huge caffeine drinker, curb that, too. It will help make the transition into the cleanse easier for you. Not that it's going to be a big system shock if you don't! But some of these foods can literally be

"I've heard so many awful things about juice cleanses: Everyone I know who has done one gains the weight right back and finds them annoying to do. But the meals on the Reboot filled me up and made me feel incredible. I had plenty of energy for my hour-and-a-half dance classes. When do you ever hear that about a juice diet?"
—*Rebecca G.*

addictive, and if you're eating boatloads of them now, you may find quitting them cold turkey a bit more difficult. Studies suggest that some of the common additives in highly processed foods cause inflammation in the body and may promote obesity—by fooling our taste buds in a way that blunts our internal satiety cues, and making us overeat. Highly processed foods are also deliberately engineered to make us crave them, lighting up the same "reward" area of the brain that drugs like cocaine do. They may linger in your system longer, too. So try to eat cleaner leading up to your Reboot.

Ditto once the three days are up and you transition back to a more normal diet (if you're not going right to the next chapter, where I show you how to use blends in your daily cooking). Try to keep eating whole plant-based foods for several days. Don't jump back to eating cheeseburgers.

When prepping for the Reboot, I also find it's best to make all four blends you'll be eating at once. Rock them out, pre-portion each one, and have them ready to go in the fridge. Then there's nothing to do for the next few days but eat and enjoy.

Let's do this.

QUICK-START INSTRUCTIONS

If you want to go ahead and begin the 3-Day Reboot right away—perhaps you've done it before and know the drill—here are the basic guidelines to follow for the next few days. More instructions follow, though, that give you more how-what-why details.

There are only five simple guidelines to remember for your 3-Day Reboot (which I also call the Blends Cleanse™):

1. Replace three meals a day with the purees in this chapter for three days. Follow the exact recipes and portion sizes, and promise me you won't skip.

2. Eat two snacks each day—and dessert. You'll find the quick-fix recipes later in this chapter.

3. Stick to the Cleanse Blend options in the meal chart below. They're designed to give you the right balance of nutrients from a variety of foods over the course of the day. If you only eat one blend, you'll miss out.

4. Go ahead and have a cup or two of coffee a day—or caffeinated tea. You can also add a splash of organic milk, unsweetened plant-based milk, and a little raw honey or Stevia. But steer clear of processed stuff like nondairy creamers and sugar (regular sugar or artificial).

5. Ditch the booze for now.

Couldn't be easier, right?

You'll find more helpful info about the guidelines below, but if you're ready to dive right in, you can just consult the meal chart that follows—and start making your blends. Either way, weigh yourself before you start the Reboot and then again on the morning of day four so you can measure your results!

DAY-BY-DAY MEAL PLAN

I've built some choices within this plan, but whatever blends you pick, be sure to mix it up so you get a good variety of nutrients. Tasty as it is, you probably don't want to eat just the Triple-Greens Cleanse Blend for seventy-two hours. This plan is designed to strike the right balance of protein, carbs, and fat over the course of the day and give you enough calories to not be hungry—yet still fast-track weight loss. Note: Recipes for the Reboot start on page 38.

BLENDS CLEANSE™ YOUR 3-DAY REBOOT

BREAKFAST
Berry Detox Shake

Or

Super-Greens Detox Shake

MID-MORNING SNACK
Maple–Sweet Potato Cleanse Blend

Or

Triple-Greens Cleanse Blend

LUNCH
Cauliflower-Chive Cleanse Blend

Or

Triple-Greens Cleanse Blend

AFTERNOON SNACK
Maple–Sweet Potato Cleanse Blend

Or

Triple-Greens Cleanse Blend

DINNER
White Bean–Rosemary Cleanse Blend

DESSERT
Cinnamon-Oat Truffle Treats

Total Calories for the Day:
Approximately 1,250

Guideline #1: Replace three meals a day with the blends in this chapter for three days. Do not miss any meals. *Especially* no blowing off breakfast. It's essential for weight loss. Many studies have shown that if you skip it, you'll overcompensate for the missed calories later in the day. According to the National Weight Control Registry, which follows more than ten thousand people who have lost at least thirty pounds and kept it off, 78 percent of the participants eat breakfast every single day. It's so crucial that the researchers point to it as a key to weight-loss success. So no making excuses that you don't have time to have a good morning meal. While there is some research questioning this idea, you have to go with your own experience. And I personally feel that if I skip it, I feel shaky, foggy, and definitely more prone to overeating. The detox shakes in this part of the plan are designed to deliver sustaining protein, fiber, and loads of antioxidants. They're much faster and more nutritious than grabbing a bagel at the deli, and definitely more diet-friendly than the chips you're going to grab at four P.M., when you're starving because you didn't eat breakfast. The blends you'll be having also make packing a lunch and snack for work infinitely easier, too.

Along with your three squares, be sure to drink plenty of water throughout the day. In addition to keeping you hydrated and your digestive system humming along, it may also speed weight loss even more. Recent research has found that sipping two 8-ounce glasses of water before meals may help you drop more pounds—and keep them off!—than if you just reduced the calories in your food, likely because good old H2O helps with satiety.

Guideline #2: Eat two snacks each day—and dessert! You might think that bypassing these extra bites will help you drop weight even faster. Not so. You need them to get enough calories, keep your metabolism up, and get all the requisite nutrients. So don't skip them! You'll only feel hangry and lousy. And trust me: Even the dessert isn't a splurge-y extra; it's actually highly nutritious and satisfying. Rather than thinking of it as snacks and treats, think of it as simply eating at six different occasions during the day (three meals, two snacks, and one dessert) and try to have something every two to three hours. It will help keep your blood sugar and insulin levels stable, thereby controlling your appetite and fending off cravings.

Remember to stick to *just* the recipes in this chapter. The next few days are about getting as much nutrition as possible—and giving your taste buds a fresh start. And definitely no outside packaged snacks, because most of them are loaded with junk. This phase is about eating as little processed food as possible and clearing your system of all that excess salt, sugar, unhealthy fat, and chemicals.

Guideline #3: Stick to the Cleanse Blend options in the meal chart on page 32. They're designed to give you the right balance of nutrients from a variety of foods over the course of the day. And be sure to mix up your meal and snack choices. If you only eat one type of blend, you'll miss out on the broader spectrum of phytonutrients.

Guideline #4: Go ahead and have a cup or two of coffee a day—or caffeinated tea. Some cleanses call for nixing it completely, but I find going moderate is the way to go. Cutting out caffeine cold turkey is literally going to be a big, fat headache that will make you less likely to stick to the plan. It's more apt to sabotage your entire cleanse than anything else. If you want to wean yourself off caffeine, give yourself more time to do it slowly, so that the withdrawal symptoms won't be so annoying.

Plus, there's good evidence that moderate consumption of coffee and tea (particularly green tea) has many health benefits. The antioxidants they contain help lower your risk for things like heart disease, type 2 diabetes, and cancer. There's even some research linking them with weight loss. And they help move things along in your G.I. tract, if you know what I mean—helping to flush toxins out faster.

Aside from these beverages, just stick with water—no fruit juices (sugar bomb!) or diet sodas. Yes, diet sodas are calorie free, but they're also loaded with chemicals. And a growing body of evidence suggests that the artificial sweeteners they contain may increase your risk of obesity, as well as affect blood sugar levels—and increase the risk of diabetes. Back away!

Guideline #5: Ditch the booze for now. Look, I love a good cocktail, too, but the fact is that alcohol is empty calories your body does not need. And while, yes, it does have some undeniable health benefits—like lowering the risk of heart disease—it also acts like liquid sugar in the body and is, technically, a toxin.

MORE SUCCESS SECRETS

✦ Eat within an hour of waking in the morning, so your blood sugar doesn't get so low you're tempted to cheat with whatever random morsel finds its way in front of you.

✦ Remember to eat something every two to three hours. You know what happens when blood sugar dips.

✦ Eat like a Buddhist. Sit down, eat slowly and mindfully, and put your spoon down between bites to give your body a chance to register the food you've eaten. You'll truly taste and enjoy your food and may feel more satisfied because of it—and need to eat less.

TRY THIS! Oats are normally processed on equipment that handles wheat products; so if you're on a gluten-free diet, look for ones that specifically say gluten free.

YOUR MASTER SHOPPING LIST

Here's a list of everything you'll need to pick up—and blend—for the 3-Day Reboot. The list is enough to make all of the blend recipes, so you may have leftovers, depending on the choices you make. Happy shopping!

FRESH PRODUCE

2 medium heads cauliflower

2 large sweet potatoes or yams

6 large carrots

1 10-ounce bag baby spinach
   (you'll need 7 cups)

1 6-ounce bag baby kale
   (you'll need 3 cups)

Broccoli, fresh or frozen
   (you'll need 4 cups florets)

1 ripe avocado

2 bananas

Fresh chives

Small bunch fresh basil or mint

Small bunch fresh rosemary

FRIDGE

1 large container plain low-fat
   Greek yogurt (or unsweetened
   plain or vanilla protein powder)

Low-fat milk or unsweetened
   plant-based milk

Small wedge Parmesan cheese

FREEZER FRUITS AND VEGETABLES

1 15-ounce bag frozen wild berries
   (blueberries, raspberries, or
   mixed berries; you'll need
   3 cups)

3 cups frozen peas

PANTRY

2 15-ounce cans (BPA-free)
   white beans, such as Great
   Northern, navy, butter, or

cannellini (You can also use
   dried beans.)

100% fruit, no-sugar-added jam

Almond butter (or Sneaky Chef
   No-Nut Butter, available at
   thesneakychef.com)
Black peppercorns (for grinding)
Chia seeds
Ground flaxseed
Ground cinnamon, ideally Ceylon
Extra-virgin olive oil

Low-sodium boxed vegetable
   broth
Pure maple syrup
Raw honey
Red pepper flakes
Rolled oats (or gluten-free oats)
Sea salt

3-DAY REBOOT RECIPES

All the recipes in this book use one of my fifteen Base Blends. You'll be using four of them for the 3-Day Reboot in this part of the plan. (See all fifteen starting on page 78.) The Base Blends are simply blitzed fruits and veggies with a little water added to help them puree down. That's it! You'll use them to create the Reboot recipes that follow; they're what I call Cleanse Blends. And even those are super-fast to put together. You're really just adding a few extra ingredients to amp up the flavors of each Base Blend. Remember to measure out portion sizes of each meal and snack and stick to the game plan. Enjoy!

If you have particular dietary requirements, check the icons by each recipe. Here's the key:

 = Gluten free

 = Low carb (contains minimal carbohydrates—no more than 10
   grams per serving)

V = Vegetarian (may include dairy, but no eggs, fish, poultry, or
   meat)

DF = Dairy free

THE BASE BLENDS

Puree each of the four Base Blends that follow to your preference—you can add a little more liquid and puree it longer in a high-powered blender or food processor if you like a super-smooth consistency. If you want more texture in your life, just blend it a bit less. (A regular blender won't work as well. It requires too much liquid to puree down and will become soupy.) Note that I call for tap water for steaming produce, but *filtered* water if it's an ingredient in a recipe that's going to be eaten.

(GF) (LC) (V) (DF)

CAULIFLOWER BASE BLEND

• Makes 6 cups •

This is the lightest of all my blends; yet since it's made with a cruciferous vegetable, it has incredible health benefits. (See page 16.) Even people who find steamed cauliflower hard on the belly can often handle this blend with no problem, because pureeing it breaks down the cell walls in a way that makes it easier to digest. Blending also makes it easier for your body to absorb cauliflower's beneficial phytonutrients. Win-win! You can totally swap in frozen cauliflower florets here, if you'd like. Just run them under hot water to thaw them a little before putting them in your blender.

10 cups cauliflower florets
  (about 2 medium heads)

Filtered water

Place a steamer basket into a large pot, pour in a few inches of tap water (make sure the water is below the bottom of the basket), and set it over high heat. Add the cauliflower and steam, covered, for 9 to 11 minutes, until fork-tender. Remove from heat and blend cooked cauliflower with ¼ cup filtered water until smooth, adding more water as necessary.

BROCCOLI-PEA-SPINACH BASE BLEND

GF V DF

• *Makes 4 cups* •

In many cases, I prefer the ease of frozen fruits and veggies, but go for the fresh, prewashed, bagged baby spinach here—it has a milder flavor. If you must use frozen (the chopped baby spinach that comes in a block), only use 1 cup for this recipe. Oh, and if you like fresh baby kale better than spinach, go ahead and swap it in.

4 cups broccoli florets, fresh or frozen

3 cups frozen sweet green peas

4 cups baby spinach

Filtered water

Place a steamer basket into a large pot, pour in a few inches of tap water (make sure the water is below the bottom of the basket), and set it over high heat. Add the broccoli and steam, covered, for about 10 minutes if fresh, or about 2 minutes if frozen, until just tender. Add the frozen peas to the basket for the last 2 minutes of steaming. Pulse the spinach in a high-powered blender a few times to reduce its volume. Add the steamed veggies along with 2 to 3 tablespoons of filtered water, and puree until smooth, adding more water as necessary.

CARROT-SWEET POTATO BASE BLEND

• Makes about 4 1/2 cups •

This blend takes a bit more time than some of the others, but I have to tell you—it's my favorite child. It works in almost anything thanks to its creamy, deliciously sweet flavor profile. Don't drive yourself crazy dicing the veggies; a rough chop is fine. Just try to make them roughly the same size so they cook evenly. Some markets do sell frozen diced sweet potatoes. If you can find these timesavers, use them. Pick up some frozen carrots, too. Then you can skip the steaming and simply flash-thaw them by pouring hot water over both veggies and go directly to the blending step. You'll need about 4 cups of frozen chopped sweet potatoes and 3 cups of frozen chopped carrots total.

2 large sweet potatoes or yams, peeled and roughly chopped

6 large carrots, peeled and roughly chopped

Filtered water

Place a steamer basket into a large pot, pour in a few inches of tap water (make sure the water is below the bottom of the basket), and set it over high heat. Add the sweet potatoes and carrots and steam, covered, for 15 to 20 minutes, until fork-tender. Blend the veggies with 2 to 3 tablespoons of filtered water until smooth, adding more water as necessary.

WHITE BEAN BASE BLEND

• Makes about 2 ¼ cups •

GF
V
DF

This recipe makes enough blend to get you through the three days of the Reboot. It's hugely versatile: It can go savory and replace mayo or cream in a recipe, or go sweet and stand in for the butter or oil in baked goods. If you'd rather use dried beans, just soak them overnight and cook according to the package directions.

2 15-ounce cans white beans, such as Great Northern, navy, butter, or cannellini, drained and rinsed

Filtered water

Blend the beans along with 2 to 3 tablespoons of filtered water until smooth, adding more water as necessary.

3-DAY REBOOT RECIPES

With the exception of the morning detox shakes, each of the recipes here takes a Base Blend and punches up the flavor—so you can eat it virtually straight up. And because the ingredients help support the detox process (see pages 23–24 for more on that), I call them Cleanse Blends. They're super-convenient, easy, and portable—so you can take lunch to the office in a to-go cup or Thermos.

BERRY DETOX SHAKE

GF
V
* DF

• *Makes 1 serving* •

This shake has it all: good fat, good protein, and good fiber. It doesn't include a Base Blend per se, because you're really just making one on the spot.

1 cup frozen wild berries (blueberries, raspberries, or mixed berries)

½ cup plain low-fat Greek yogurt (or 1 scoop unsweetened plain or vanilla protein powder)

1 tablespoon ground flaxseed (or 1 teaspoon chia seeds)

1 cup loosely packed baby spinach

1 cup loosely packed baby kale

¼ ripe avocado

⅛ teaspoon ground cinnamon

1 to 2 teaspoons raw honey or pure maple syrup

1 cup cold filtered water

4 ice cubes

Place all of the ingredients into a high-powered blender and puree until smooth. Serve in a tall glass.

Nutrition facts: 279 calories; 9 g fat; 92 mg sodium; 38 g carbs; 13 g fiber; 17 g sugar; 15 g protein

* *(if using dairy-free protein powder)*

SUPER-GREENS DETOX SHAKE

• Makes 1 serving •

GF
V
DF *

This shake is my version of a green drink, only with loads of filling protein and fiber. Try this hack to make your A.M. prep take thirty seconds: Put all of the ingredients *except* the frozen fruit and ice in the blender and stash it in the fridge before you go to bed. In the morning, add the remaining ingredients and blend until smooth.

½ banana, ideally frozen

1 cup baby kale or baby
  spinach

1 tablespoon ground flaxseed

¼ ripe avocado

⅛ teaspoon ground cinnamon

½ cup plain low-fat Greek
  yogurt (or 1 scoop
  unsweetened plain or vanilla
  protein powder)

1 to 2 teaspoons raw honey or
  pure maple syrup

1 ½ cups filtered water

4 or 5 ice cubes

Place all of the ingredients into a high-powered blender and puree until smooth. Serve in a tall glass.

Nutrition facts: 268 calories; 9 g fat; 62 mg sodium; 37 g carbs; 8 g fiber; 20 g sugar; 15 g protein

(if using dairy-free protein powder)

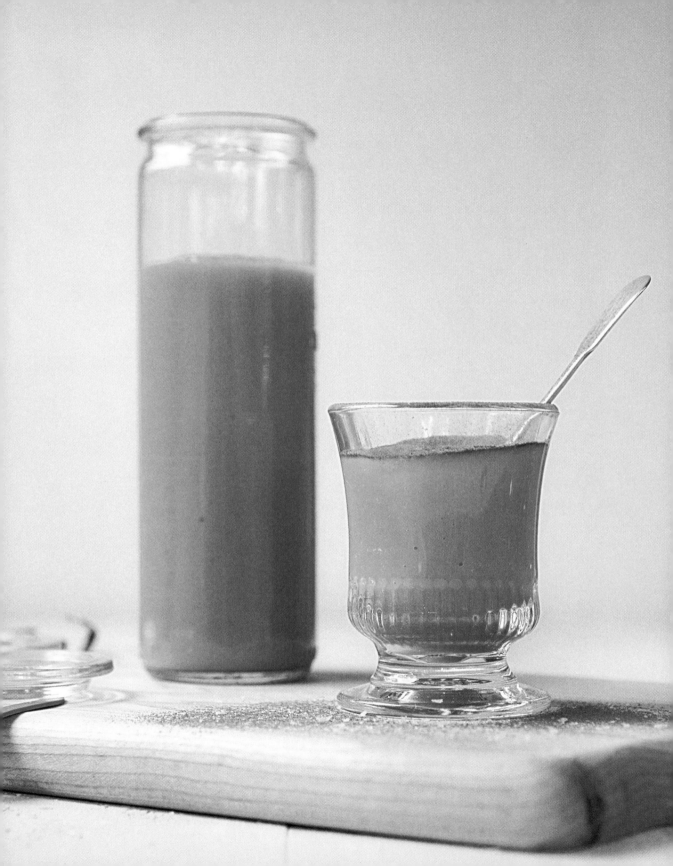

MAPLE-SWEET POTATO CLEANSE BLEND

• *Makes 1 serving* •

I would eat this morning, noon, and night if I could. Honestly! It tastes so good—sweet and soothing—like a virtuous pie filling.

1 ½ cups **Carrot–Sweet Potato Base Blend** (page 40)

2 teaspoons extra-virgin olive oil

1 to 2 teaspoons pure maple syrup

Sea salt

Ground cinnamon (optional)

Warm the blend and the oil in a small saucepan. Add the salt and cinnamon, if using, to taste, and serve.

Nutrition facts: 247 calories; 10 g fat; 150 mg sodium; 40 g carbs; 7 g fiber; 17 g sugar; 3 g protein

CAULIFLOWER-CHIVE
CLEANSE BLEND

• Makes 1 serving •

I love faux mashed potatoes, made by substituting super-light, healthy cauli-flower for starchy spuds. This is my riff on that original idea. The chives are key flavor enhancers, but there are lots of other things you can add for variety, such as fresh parsley or thyme or a little grated garlic or fresh ginger.

2 cups **Cauliflower Base Blend** (page 38)

2 tablespoons low-fat milk or unsweetened plant-based milk

2 teaspoons extra-virgin olive oil

1 tablespoon chopped fresh chives

Sea salt and freshly ground black pepper

Warm the blend, milk, and oil in a small sauce-pan. Add the chives, season to taste with salt and pepper, and serve.

Nutrition facts: 180 calories; 10 g fat; 122 mg sodium; 20 g carbs; 9 g fiber; 8 g sugar; 8 g protein

(if using plant-based milk)

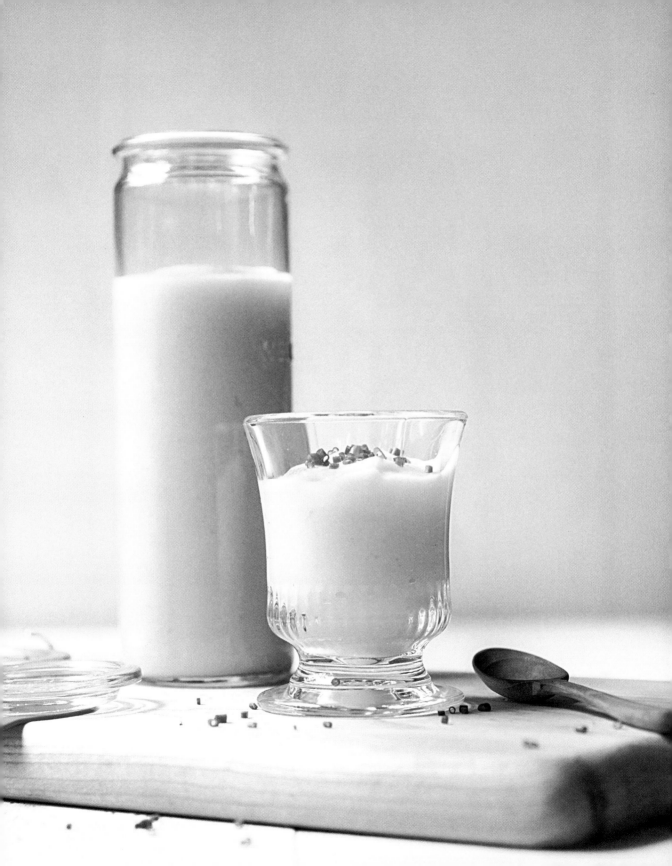

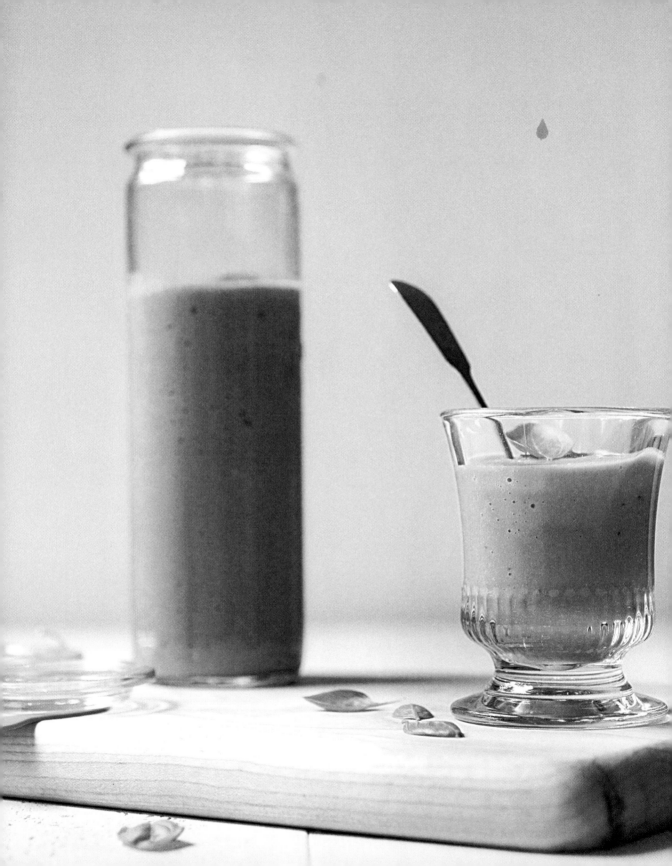

TRIPLE-GREENS CLEANSE BLEND

GF V DF

• *Makes 1 serving* •

This simple recipe contains a trifecta of greens and fresh herbs that make the whole dish sparkle. The Brits eat a version of this called "mushy peas," which are delicious but swim in butter and are cooked so long much of the nutrition is lost. Mine has a much brighter, fresher flavor.

1 cup **Broccoli-Pea-Spinach Base Blend** (page 39)

2 teaspoons extra-virgin olive oil

1 tablespoon chopped fresh basil (or 1 teaspoon chopped fresh mint)

Sea salt

Warm the blend and the oil in a small saucepan. Stir in the herbs, season with salt to taste, and serve.

Nutrition facts: 163 calories; 9 g fat; 135 mg sodium; 15 g carbs; 4 g fiber; 4 g sugar; 7 g protein

WHITE BEAN–ROSEMARY CLEANSE BLEND

• Makes 1 serving •

This soup is a favorite of almost everyone who has done my Reboot. It is creamy, warm, and filling—a great way to end the day. The fragrant rosemary takes it to a whole other level and is incredibly good for you. The herb improves digestion, has anti-inflammatory properties, and stimulates your immune system.

½ cup **White Bean Base Blend** (page 41)

1 cup low-sodium vegetable broth

1 teaspoon extra-virgin olive oil

1 tablespoon minced fresh rosemary

1 tablespoon freshly grated Parmesan cheese

Red pepper flakes

Sea salt and freshly ground black pepper

Whisk the blend, broth, and oil together in a pot over medium heat. Stir in the rosemary and Parmesan. Season with red pepper flakes and salt and pepper to taste and serve.

Nutrition facts: **223 calories; 7 g fat; 170 mg sodium; 28 g carbs; 8 g fiber; 1 g sugar; 12 g protein**

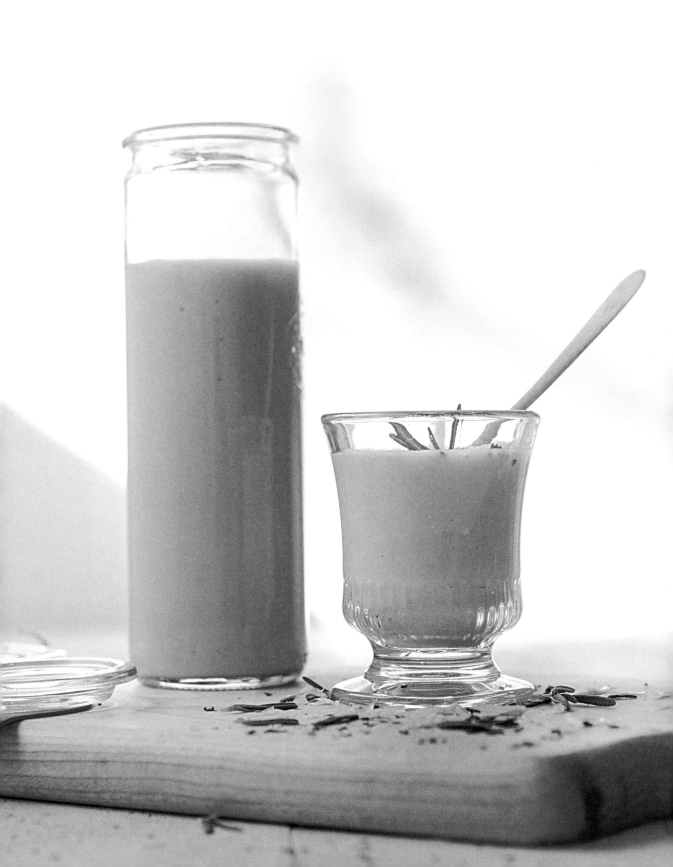

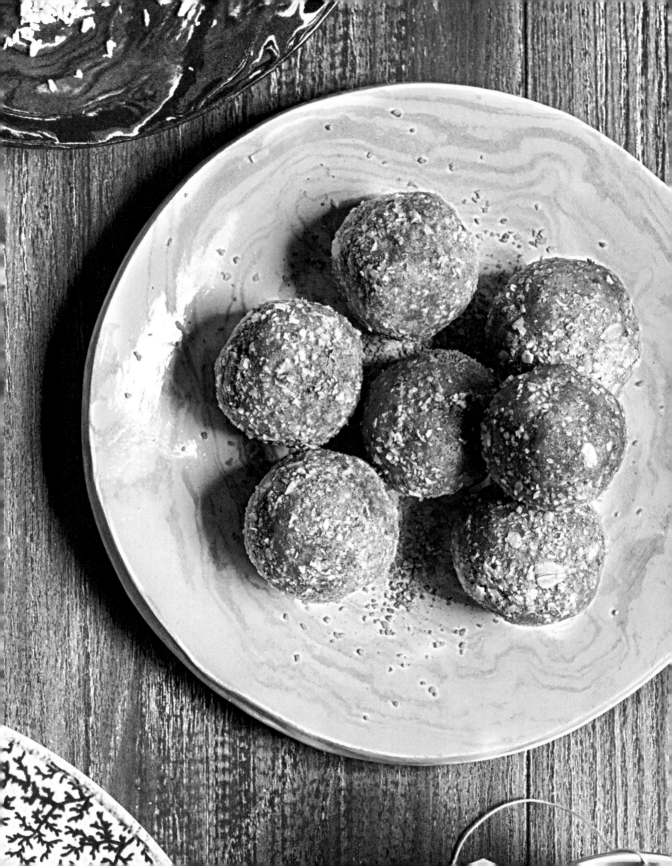

CINNAMON-OAT TRUFFLE TREATS

Makes 8 servings • Serving size: 2 truffles

That's right: dessert! On a cleanse! And who knew something packed with healthy ingredients could taste so decadent? No wonder people are obsessed with these, myself included. I have them in my freezer at all times. The crew on the photo shoot for this book called them "energy bites," and we had to keep making more because they kept disappearing. Freezing them makes the truffle treats even better, and forces you to slow down and savor them longer—so they seem even more satisfying. Check out the other varieties of these treats on pages 246 and 247.

6 tablespoons **White Bean Base Blend** (page 41)

½ cup almond butter (or Sneaky Chef No-Nut Butter)

1 tablespoon 100% fruit, no-sugar-added jam

2 tablespoons ground flaxseed

½ cup finely ground rolled oats, divided (or gluten-free oats)

⅓ teaspoon ground cinnamon

Pinch of sea salt

On a plate, mix the blend, almond butter, jam, flaxseed, and 2 tablespoons of the oats until well combined. On another plate, mix the remaining oats, with the cinnamon and salt. Use a melon baller or measuring spoon to make tablespoon-size balls of the blend mixture. Roll the truffles in the cinnamon-oat mixture. Serve right away, or place the truffles in a container and freeze for at least 30 minutes before serving.

Nutrition facts (per serving) : 144 calories; 11 g fat; 6 mg sodium; 11 g carbs; 2 g fiber; 1 g sugar; 4 g protein

* *(if using gluten-free oats)*

NOW, ABOUT THE REST OF YOUR DAY …
GET SOME EXERCISE!

We can't talk health and weight loss without also talking about exercise. As you know, what you eat is only one part of that equation. So try to break a sweat for at least thirty minutes, every day. I'm a big fan of interval training, where you alternate moderate-intensity exercise with periods when you really push it. A study in the *Journal of Strength and Conditioning Research* found that interval training burns *44 percent* more calories than doing moderate steady-state cardio or strength training for the same amount of time. And Australian researchers discovered that interval training is also better at reducing body fat—particularly belly fat (woo-hoo!). In the study, they compared three groups of people: one that did intervals, one that did the same amount of steady-state exercise, and one that did no exercise. The latter two groups actually gained a little body fat over the fifteen-week study, while the interval exercisers reduced their total body fat by 11 percent and their abdominal fat by 10 percent. Part of the reason has to do with what's known as the "afterburn" effect. During the go-all-out intense intervals, your body works anaerobically, which amps up your calorie-burning power even *after* you stop exercising. Try running for thirty seconds to one minute, then walking briskly for two to three minutes and repeating those intervals for at least thirty minutes.

If you're a beginner and the idea of intense exercise feels like too much, start out with the new *moderate* type of interval training, switching moderate-intensity exercises (a six or seven on a scale of one to ten, with ten being the hardest you can work) with easy ones. You can use the same basic routine above of walking briskly for one minute, then slowing down for two minutes and repeating the intervals for at least thirty minutes.

It's also important to strength-train a couple days a week to build lean muscle—which burns more calories all day long than the same amount of body fat. Don't be afraid of weights and don't forget to work all your major muscle groups! Not sure what to do? With so many amazing free apps and online toning routines, you can't play dumb on that one.

Make an effort to simply move more during the day, too: Pace around while you're on a conference call, or set an alarm and walk around the block every hour or so. Studies have declared sitting the new smoking. Being chair-bound for five hours or more a day increases your risk for "sitting disease," a term that refers to all the health problems that long periods of inactivity can cause—including obesity, high blood pressure, diabetes, cancer, and even depression. And, yes, research shows that sitting most of the day puts you at the same risk for heart attack as someone who smokes. Going to the gym is great, but it's not enough to tick off your activity box. Moving more throughout the day, experts say, is the real measure of good health. So aim to get up and do something for five to ten minutes of every hour. Research shows this small amount of activity is enough to stave off the metabolic idling that happens when you're sedentary. It actually changes hormone levels in your body in a way that lessens your risk for all of those sitting-related problems.

OK, NOW WHAT?

Once you've dropped those first few pounds and are feeling lighter and more energized, turn to the next chapter and start phase two of the journey. I'll show you how to incorporate blends into your everyday cooking. It's the linchpin for maintaining good nutrition and making sure the weight you've lost *stays* lost. If you need to take any time off between now and the next phase, remember to keep eating clean, whole foods like the ones your body has become accustomed to over the past three days.

ASK MISSY

Here are some things I'm often asked about the Reboot, and how to handle them.

Do I have to eat everything?

I get this question a lot, and my answer is: Try to! Otherwise, you may feel too hungry and fall off the wagon later on. You may also not get enough calories. I know that it might seem like a lot of food—filling food—but if you scope out the calorie counts you'll see that they're pretty low. Nix a meal or snack and you might actually fight your weight-loss efforts, rather than fast-track them. You can space the food out as you wish, though. So if you're not hungry for your mid-morning snack, for example, you can save it for whenever you do want it.

What if I'm hungry?

I can count the number of times I've heard this on one hand (see above). But if you really need a little extra something, go ahead and have a half cup of any of the Cleanse Blends. Or have a cup of low-sodium broth or bone broth—a current obsession of mine. Here's my recipe:

BONE BROTH

Chicken bones from 1 whole, cooked chicken	2 teaspoons sea salt
2 chopped carrots	Enough filtered water to cover all of the ingredients
2 chopped stalks celery	2 tablespoons cider vinegar or freshly squeezed lemon juice (which helps extract nutrients from the bones)
1 chopped medium onion	

In a large stockpot, combine all the ingredients and bring the soup to a boil over high heat, then reduce the heat to low, partially cover (leave just a crack open), and simmer very gently for 8 to 12 hours. Check the soup occasionally. Skim any foam from the surface and add water if need to keep the ingredients covered. Strain the broth and discard the chicken bones and vegetables. Store for up to 5 days in the fridge or 3 months in the freezer. The chilled broth should look gelatin-like. Note: If you're nervous about leaving the pot on the stove for that long, there are recipes online for doing it in a slow cooker.

"I never felt hungry, everything was super-tasty, and my energy was through the roof. The portability was key, too. It was so easy to pack up my meals and snacks and bring them to work with me. Such a doable diet!"

—Amy G.

If I miss a meal or snack should I double up at the next one?

Yes, that works. It's important not to eat too few calories, otherwise your weight-loss efforts will backfire. You'll feel too hungry and overcompensate later and your metabolism may suffer.

If I'm really in a pinch—say, traveling for work—and can't have one of the blends, what do I do?

Have a small container of low-fat Greek yogurt and some berries in place of the breakfast shake, if you must. Or have a cup of a broth-based vegetable-loaded soup in place of a meal (not the super-salty stuff that comes in a can, though; I'm talking fresh and clean!).

How are your blends better than, say, baby food—which is also pureed fruits and veggies?

There's a world of difference between wholesome homemade blends and jarred, processed food. Baby food is pasteurized, a process that kills enzymes that help with digestion and destroys some (or most) of the vitamins and phytonutrients in the produce. My blends aren't heated to oblivion—so you get more nutrition. Plus, fresh tastes so much better! There's no comparison.

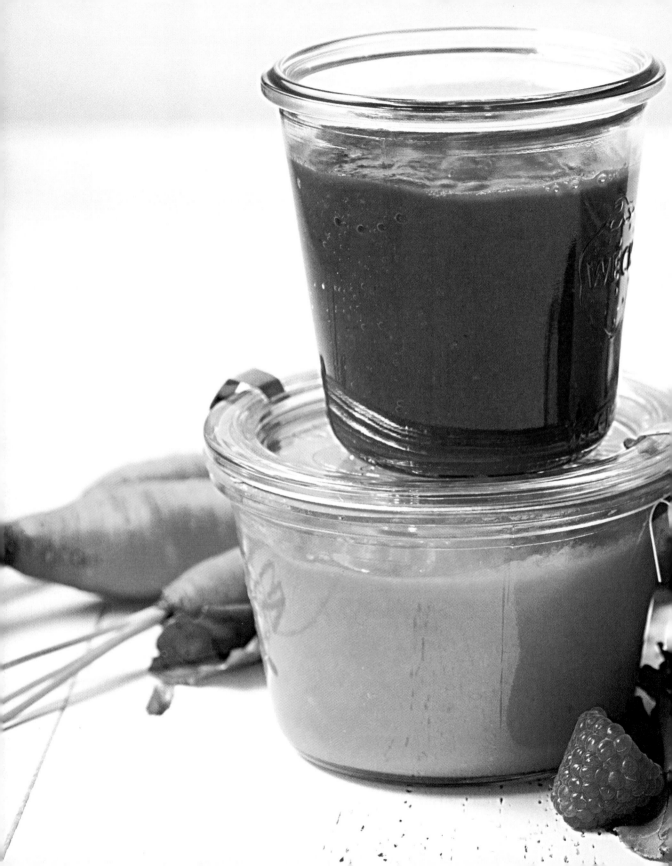

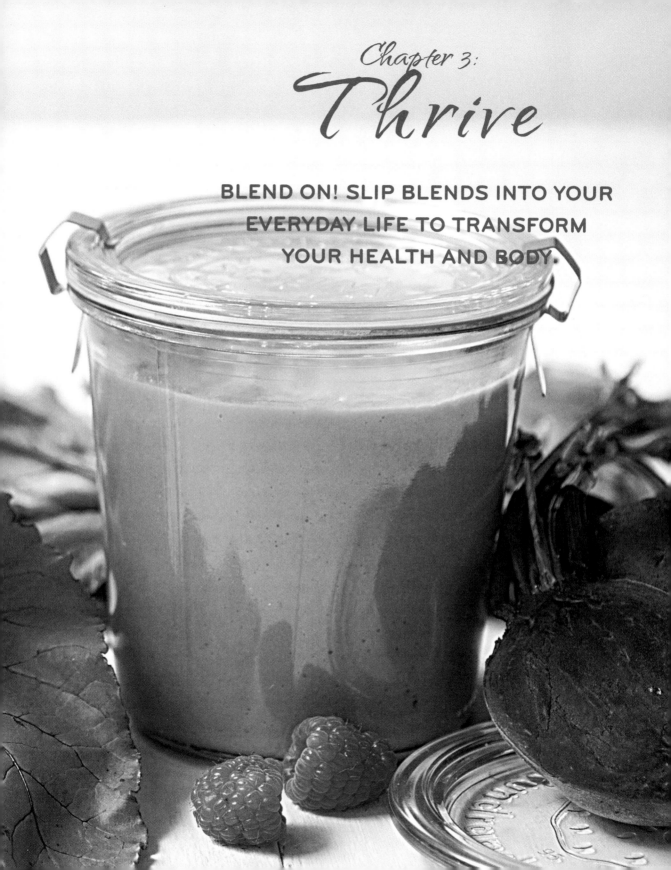

Chapter 3:
Thrive

BLEND ON! SLIP BLENDS INTO YOUR
EVERYDAY LIFE TO TRANSFORM
YOUR HEALTH AND BODY.

Welcome to the second part of the plan. How are you feeling these days? Refreshed? Energized? A whole lot lighter? Let's keep it that way! Now that you've gotten used to prepping and using my blends from the Reboot, I want to show you how to incorporate them into your everyday life—to help you maintain both a healthy weight and good nutrition. Because you've already had a taste of how blending works, the transition should be seamless. Not so with juice diets! Once you're done, that's it: You're left adrift with no direction, which means you're bound to fall into your old eating habits again. No wonder the weight always goes right back on. My blends allow you to shift from the Reboot to a forever way of cooking and eating. It's the "lifestyle" that experts are always touting as the key to long-term success.

"I can't believe I can 'have my cake and eat it too!' No more low-carb dieting for me. Now I can enjoy all the foods I'd previously given up thanks to this incredibly easy way of cooking!" —Risa G.

Now, my blends go from being a delicious food you enjoy almost on their own, to an incredibly versatile tool—an ingredient that can transform your favorite foods into healthier versions of themselves, without you even noticing the difference. Check the numbers: Studies show that swapping purees (or blends) for some of the more caloric ingredients in foods can help you eat 357 calories fewer each day, on average—without feeling any less satisfied—so you'll continue to lose weight, if you still need to. The same research also shows that adding blends to meals will up your fruit and veg intake by an average of two servings a day. Pretty great, huh?

By adding blends to everything you make—whether it's a recipe in this book or your mom's famous lasagna—you can also satisfy the inner bad girl we all have. Because the truth is, as righteous as we want to be, we want it all—and I'm here to give it all back to you. With my blends, you can literally have your chocolate cake and eat it, too. Fascinating fact: Research shows that humans are hardwired to counterbalance their "good" choices (like tossing a big bunch of broccoli into your shopping cart) with "bad" ones (grabbing a bowling ball–size chocolate chip muffin). And the more good decisions you make, the more tempting the bad ones become. Psychologists call it the "licensing effect" and you can't willpower your way out of it. Now you don't have to! By using my blends in your cooking, you can strike the perfect balance between the good (low-cal and loaded with phytonutrients!) and the bad (and it's a *whoopie pie*!), which makes for a way of eating you can commit to for life and actually win at. It was a completely life-changing revelation to me—and I hope it is for you, too!

"This is the easiest way to incorporate more veggies and fruits into your daily life. Before I started doing blends, I'd wake up with the best intentions, but never make my goal. With Missy's blends, I almost never miss getting all the good stuff in every single day!" —Laura K.

2 SUCCESS SECRETS TO BLENDING FOR LIFE

All the details on blending follows—and trust me, it's easier than you can imagine. And while this part of the plan doesn't have any hard-and-fast rules to follow, I do have a few pointers that will set you up for success and keep the scale digits as low as you want—for good. Here goes:

1. *Have at least two Base Blends in your fridge at all times.* That way, you'll be more likely to *use* them. Mine are front-and-center in the fridge, so they're staring me in the face every time I open it. There's something powerful about seeing them every time you open your fridge that will help keep you on track.

(And there's actually research that shows you're more likely to grab something out of the refrigerator if it's at eye level in the middle of the shelf.)

Don't forget the beautiful jars, too! Weck or mason jars make great storage containers, and your blends will look uber-cool in them. Another tip: Stock your fridge and pantry with blend ingredients, so you'll always be able to whip one up in minutes if you run out. Time is your biggest deterrent when it comes to eating healthy—so stack the deck in your favor.

I find the Carrot–Sweet Potato and White Bean blends to be the most versatile, so those would be two good ones to have on hand; but go with whichever you like best.

2. *Use your blends in everything you make!* For starters, cook from this book. It's a way to keep calories down without even trying. In fact, one of the challenges I found developing recipes for this book is that often the blends made the calories so low that I had to find ways to get them up a bit. *That's* telling. (Even though they're just as filling as their higher-cal counterparts, I didn't want to scare people off by seeing such low numbers.)

Not only will you shave more calories off your day—in a totally imperceptible way—it's also more foolproof than trying to track calories on your own. Studies show most people are terrible at guesstimating daily calories. What's more, we tend to underestimate how much we're actually eating. With my meals, the numbers are all right in front of you and you know you can pick any breakfast, lunch, and dinner you want and feel confident that you're getting the nutrition you need while staying well within your caloric parameters. And with my recipes, you'll also get more nutrients, so your body will work better for you.

This is not about committing to a certain diet. It's about making it extremely easy to eat better, while still enjoying the foods Americans want to eat—from pizza to cookies. And there's no reason not to! If you have a craving for something, check the book before you order out, because odds are, it's in here. And if you want help making your favorite dish healthier by adding a blend, email me at info@thesneakychef.com. I revamp recipes for people all the time.

SWAP IN BLENDS, SAVE MAJOR CALORIES!

Take a look at how my recipes stack up against traditionally made versions from some common chain restaurants (per serving).

MY RECIPES	TRADITIONAL RECIPES	
"No More Muffin Top!" *Blueberry Muffin Tops* 181 calories 6 grams fat 12 grams sugar	*Muffin Top* 350 calories 13 grams fat 30 grams sugar	You get half the calories and 3 times less sugar (none of which comes from refined sugar).
Curried Chicken Salad– *Stuffed Pitas* 274 calories 5 grams fat 159 milligrams sodium 5 grams fiber	*Curried Chicken Salad* *Sandwich (from a popular* *chain restaurant)* 470 calories 27 grams fat 770 milligrams sodium 2 grams fiber	This version has far fewer calories, about 5 times less fat and salt, and more than double the amount of fiber as the traditional mayo-loaded lunch offering has.
Meaty Mushroom *Bolognese* 348 calories 10 grams fat 203 milligrams sodium	*Spaghetti Bolognese with* *Mushrooms* 930 calories 37 grams fat 999 milligrams sodium	Mine has nearly ⅓ the calories and 4 times less fat—and *waaay* less salt.

READY-MADE PUREES

You can lean on these guys if you find yourself in a pinch, or are short on time, and don't have a homemade blend on hand. But remember: Just because they're a similar consistency doesn't mean they're as good for you. They aren't as unprocessed and nutritious as my blends. But you can use them in recipes in just the same way—to add vitamins and minerals and take down the overall calories.

Swap in: Guacamole	*For:* Sweet Pea Base Blend
Swap in: Hummus	*For:* Chickpea-Zucchini Base Blend
Swap in: White bean hummus	*For:* White Bean Base Blend
Swap in: Canned or frozen squash puree *and* no-sugar-added applesauce	*For:* Butternut Squash–Apple Base Blend
Swap in: Canned 100% pumpkin puree	*For:* Pumpkin Base Blend
Swap in: Vegetarian refried beans *and* blueberry organic baby food	*For:* Black Bean–Blueberry–Baby Kale Base Blend
Swap in: Organic baby food—a blend with spinach and berries	*For:* Blueberry–Baby Spinach or Mixed Berry–Baby Kale Base Blends
Swap in: Canned beets, mashed	*For:* Beet Base Blend
Swap in: Organic squeezie fruit-and-veggie pouches, like Mamma Chia	*For:* Many of the blends, depending on the flavor combos. (And it's okay if it has an extra ingredient in the mix.)

When you're *not* making one of my recipes, aim to use blends as much as you can in your own cooking. And don't be intimidated. They mix into pretty much everything you eat. Here are a whole bunch of ideas. You don't have to use a lot in each dish, either. I always say that a little here and a little there really adds up over the course of the day. Add even a tablespoon several times a day and you'll wind up having ¼ cup—which is the equivalent of an entire extra serving of fruits and veg. (Remember: Blends are concentrated and count for at least double the whole produce.) Not only will you get more nutrition into your life, you'll also be replacing ingredients that aren't as good for you, like unhealthy fats. Take a look at all the ways you can use them, and experiment! Once you get the hang of it, adding them will become second nature.

TRY THIS! Never let another too-ripe banana go to waste. Peel it and throw it in a baggie in the freezer. You'll always find a use for frozen bananas in smoothies, desserts—everything. Peeling them first is key! I recently had to wrestle the peel off a frozen one and it was a nightmare.

40 WAYS TO SLIP BLENDS INTO YOUR EVERYDAY MEALS

Green Base Blends (Broccoli-Pea-Spinach, Sweet Pea–Baby Kale and Sweet Pea)
1. Mix them into green things, like guac and pesto.
2. Add them into dishes with ground meat, like meatballs and chili.
3. Stir them into gravy.
4. Add them to your morning omelet or frittata.
5. Put a bit in your green drink.

Purple Base Blends (Blueberry–Baby Spinach, Mixed Berry–Baby Kale, and Black Bean–Blueberry–Baby Kale)
6. Use them to replace half the fat and sugar in chocolaty baked goods, like brownies or chocolate cake.
7. Mix them into meaty dishes, like tacos or burgers.

8. Add one of the berry-based blends to smoothie bowls or breakfast shakes.

Orange Base Blends (Carrot–Sweet Potato, Butternut Squash–Apple, and Pumpkin)

9. Stir them into soups to add creaminess—without the cream.
10. Use them to replace half the fat and sugar in baked goods, like muffins.
11. Ditto breakfast items such as pancakes and waffles.
12. Mix them into nut butters.
13. Stir them into any red sauces, like marinara or pizza sauces.
14. Add them to replace some of the cheese in recipes like mac and cheese or quesadillas.
15. Mix them into store-bought hummus.
16. Add them to condiments, like ketchup and mustard.
17. Try them in salad dressings.
18. Use them in brown gravies.
19. Whisk them into soups.
20. Doctor up prepared baked beans with them.
21. Mix them into meaty dishes, like meatloaf.

White Base Blends (Chickpea-Zucchini, White Bean, and Cauliflower)

22. Use them in tuna or chicken salad in place of some or all of the mayo.
23. Same with creamy side dishes like coleslaw.
24. Add them to Mexican dishes, like tacos and burritos.
25. Try them in Chinese sauces, like traditional brown or peanut sauces.
26. Replace the cream in recipes with them; they add the same velvety effect.
27. Mix them half and half with salad dressings, like ranch or blue cheese.
28. Use them in white sauces, in place of some of the butter, cream, or cheese.
29. Add them to all kinds of dips.
30. Lighten up mashed potatoes with Cauliflower Blend or Chickpea-Zucchini Blend.
31. Try White Bean Blend in sweet baked goods.
32. Stir them into polenta.

33. Mix them into your biscuit or cornbread recipes.
34. Add them into your scrambled eggs or omelets.

Red Base Blends (Raspberry-Beet, Raspberry, Beet)

35. Try them in smoothie bowls.
36. Use them in baked foods—especially chocolate dishes, like red velvet cupcakes—to replace half the fat and sugar.
37. Add them to drinks, like shakes and lemonades—or just add to seltzer water.
38. Stir them into barbecue or teriyaki sauces.
39. Whisk them into fruit-based sauces for meat dishes.
40. Cut sweeter-tasting salad dressings with them.

By using two of your blends during the day, the benefits can be pretty mind blowing. Go through a half cup each of my Mixed Berry–Baby Kale and Broccoli-Pea-Spinach Base Blends, for example, and you'll get the equivalent of two servings of fruit and three servings of veg—as well as seven different types of produce with a wide range of vitamins, minerals, and phytonutrients. That's *on top of* the produce that's actually in the meals

HOW TO USE A CUP OF BLEND A DAY

✦ I wake up and brush my teeth with Broccoli-Pea-Spinach Base Blend (Kidding! Just making sure you're paying attention.)

✦ I add Mixed Berry–Baby Kale Base Blend to whole grain pancakes for the whole fam.

✦ I warm up Broccoli-Pea-Spinach Base Blend and have it as a morning snack with a little chopped basil stirred in.

✦ I mix a little avocado with Broccoli-Pea-Spinach Base Blend and spread it on my turkey sandwich at lunchtime instead of mayo.

✦ I stir a spoonful of Greek yogurt and a touch of raw honey into Mixed Berry–Baby Kale Base Blend for an afternoon snack.

✦ I add Broccoli-Pea-Spinach Base Blend to store-bought pesto and toss with whole grain pasta for dinner.

✦ I use Mixed Berry–Baby Kale Base Blend as a base for make-'em-in-a-flash brownies (check out the recipe on page 243).

SKINNIFIED SNACKS

Check out how many calories you can save eating my between-meal bites.

MY RECIPES	TRADITIONAL RECIPES	
Crab and Artichoke Dip 58 calories 1 g fat	*Crab and Artichoke Dip* 220 calories 18 grams fat	This dip has 74 percent fewer calories, thanks to nixing all that mayo.
4 P.M. Protein Cookie 141 calories 5 grams protein	*Oatmeal Raisin Cookie* 180 calories 2 grams protein	My version has more than double the sustaining protein—in fact, this snack has as much protein as an egg.
5-a-Day Brownies 131 calories 7 grams fat 9 grams sugar	*Commercially Prepared Brownies* 226 calories 9 grams fat 21 grams sugar	You get a sweet (and nutritious!) treat with half the calories and sugar. Plus, this one's sweetened with healthy, all-natural ingredients, not refined sugar. Yum!

TRY THIS! Frozen grapes and orange slices make an amazing snack. You eat them more slowly and there's something incredibly satisfying about them; it's like having little bites of sorbet, only much healthier.

you make. You'll be a lean, mean, healthy superstar. And your body will feel better and well nourished. I describe how I do it in the sidebar on page 67.

MORE SUCCESS SECRETS

✦ Continue having snacks in your life—including a sweet bite after dinner. If you go more than two to three hours you're going to get ravenous and over-eat. You can DIY, of course, but if you're trying to drop more pounds, eating my snacks might be your best bet (see chart at left).

✦ Stay off the processed foods and sugary drinks—even the diet stuff. Sugar and refined grains are known to not only promote weight gain, but also up your risk for heart disease and diabetes. And emerging research suggests that artificial sweeteners may have the same effect. By this point, though, many people who have done the Reboot find they don't crave or want them, anyway! Their palate has shifted to a newer, cleaner preference for food. If you need a little somethin' in your Greek yogurt or coffee, these are your best options: pure maple syrup, raw honey, Stevia or other

5 WAYS TO TELL IF A FOOD IS TOO PROCESSED

Yes, there are exceptions to these rules—raw honey, for example, has a long shelf life, and isn't highly processed—but generally, if an item has one or more of the following things, then it's overly monkeyed with. Move along!

1. It has a long ingredients list. As in, more than a handful of them.

2. It contains ingredients that don't grow, walk, fly, or swim, like artificial colors or sweeteners, chemicals, preservatives, or hydrogenated oils.

3. It has a crazy-long shelf life. (Why hello there, Twinkies!)

4. It contains refined flour (look for the words "enriched" or "bleached flour").

5. It's got loads of added sugars, including high-fructose corn syrup, or loads of salt (more than about 400 milligrams per serving).

natural sugar substitute, dates, and bananas. The more processed ones to avoid: white table sugar, brown sugar, sugar substitutes like Splenda, and corn syrup.

✦ Sip lots of water. There is no set amount to aim for; that whole eight glasses thing is actually a myth. But being well hydrated will help all the amazing fiber you're eating pass through your system more easily, so toxins clear your system quickly, too. And according to a CDC study, 43 percent of Americans don't drink enough water. Drink up. H2O is also key for keeping your energy up and staying focused, and it has even been shown to help with weight loss. If your pee is pale yellow, you're good. You can make your water infinitely more interesting by trying one of these flavoring ideas: strawberry and lime, cucumber and lime, raspberry and lime, watermelon, watermelon and basil, and mango. If you want more flavor, toss a small amount in your glass and muddle with the back of a wooden spoon. They're all totally delicious and calorie free!

✦ Check in with how you feel. A lot of people never really take a moment to consider how their own body is feeling. How's your energy level? Are you having fewer food cravings? Do you feel more clear-headed? This is a great way to make sure things are still working for you—because it's not all about how much you weigh, it's about how you feel overall!

TRY THIS! Stick to heart-healthy fats, like extra-virgin olive oil or coconut oil, as much as possible.

WANT TO FAST-TRACK WEIGHT LOSS?

Yes, the pounds should keep coming off once you start incorporating blends into your daily diet. But if you want to speed up that process, I've found it works best to replace your two regular snacks with the blends in the chart that follows until you reach your goal weight. Research shows that we're eating between meals more than ever these days, and a very high percentage of the excess calories in our diets come from those snacks. The average American now eats a whopping *580 calories* worth of snacks a day—220 more than compared to a few decades ago. And they account for 25 percent of our daily calories.

Not only that, but *what* we're nibbling tends to be highly processed—the kind of foods that studies have linked to poorer health and weight gain. By replacing those *meh* obesogenic snacks with nutrient-charged blends, you'll retrain your taste buds to crave fresh, wholesome foods—not the ones that have been engineered to trigger your "bliss point," as the food industry refers to it, and make you crave more, more, more of these nutrient-void, processed salty/sweet/fatty snacks.

"Transitioning to having blends in place of snacks is such a fresh idea. And it's so appealing and doable—I freaked out over how amazing the blends were. This is pure, real, true food that is still unbelievably good. And there's such a wide variety that you never get bored."
—*Lisa J.*

I'm no registered dietician here, but just do the math: Replace your between-meal bites with two of mine and you could save between 200 and 300 calories a day—deliciously and effortlessly—which equals about an extra five-pound weight loss in two weeks *just* from switching out your snacks. In addition to that, you'll be eating yummy meals that further reduce your daily caloric intake in a meaningful way.

I also find that snacks are much more flexible than meals in terms of swapping in something else—which means you're much more apt to stick with it. No one ever takes their favorite low-cal dish to a breakfast meeting or dinner party, and a weight-loss plan needs to be uber-usable and practical—otherwise it can't be effective.

Below is a list of some blend choices. Some of them make two servings—so you can have half for your morning snack and half in the afternoon. Just be sure to get two of them every day. P.S., while you're doing this, if you're craving dessert, make sure it's one from the book.

RECIPE NAME	BLEND IT USES	PAGE
Savory Blends		
½ cup Triple-Greens Cleanse Blend (makes 2 snack-size servings) 82 calories	*Broccoli-Pea-Spinach Base Blend*	90
¾ cup White Bean–Rosemary Cleanse Blend (makes 2 snack-size servings) 112 calories	*White Bean Base Blend*	83
½ cup Warm Green Basil Blend (makes 2 snack-size servings) 112 calories	*Broccoli-Pea-Spinach Base Blend*	90
½ cup Thai-Style Blend (makes 2 snack-size servings) 124 calories	*Sweet Pea Base Blend*	92
½ cup Tex-Mex Blend (makes 2 snack-size servings) 128 calories	*Black Bean–Blueberry–Baby Kale Base Blend*	100
Bean and Goat Cheese Blend 115 calories	*Chickpea-Zucchini Base Blend*	82
Rosemary–White Bean Blend 139 calories	*White Bean Base Blend*	83
Cauliflower-Chive Blend 105 calories	*Cauliflower Base Blend*	84

ASK MISSY

My blender and I have been spinning for more than ten years, so if you get stuck, I may be able to help.

How do I know how much blend to add to my own recipes?
In baking, start by replacing half the fat in a recipe with a blend; for dishes like soups and sauces, replace all the cream and oil or butter. For other recipes— meatloaf, pancakes, pasta, sauces, etc.—start small by adding a few tablespoons of blend and work your way up from there. You can always add more, but you can't take it out!

All of a sudden, my weight loss stalled. What's going on?
Do a little dietary sleuthing to figure out what's going on: Keep a food diary for a few days and write down everything you eat or drink—including portion sizes. I do it all the time and it's a real eye-opener! You may have gotten portion creep, where a half cup of pasta burgeons into a cup. Measuring out your servings for a few days might help. Or maybe you're doing the BLT thing: bites, licks, and tastes that you take while prepping food for yourself or your family. They can add up to several hundred extra calories a day. Also, make sure you're eating *enough*. Believe it or not, eating too little can slow weight loss. Here's a simple formula I've found helpful for figuring out the number of calories you need to keep the scale moving down:

1. Multiply your current weight by 10 (for women) or 11 (men).

2. Add 20 percent to that number if you don't exercise; 30 percent if you exercise sometimes; 40 percent if you are moderately active and 50 percent if you work out regularly.

3. Shave 500 to 1,000 calories from that number through either diet or exercise and you'll lose weight.

What if I start to gain some of the weight back?

Log all your food and workouts and see where you might be going off the rails a little—then use that info to rein yourself back in. Make sure you're sipping plenty of water, too. It's easy to mistake thirst for hunger and wind up eating when you really don't need the extra calories. And if you've been eating out more than usual, try to make more meals at home; the average restaurant meal contains 1,500 calories! Sit down—with a knife and fork—before you eat, too. It prevents mindless eating on your feet. I also like to weigh myself frequently, so I can catch a small uptick in weight before it goes from two pounds to ten. Research shows that this strategy is a key to long-term weight-loss success.

"Any time I overdo the refined carbs and sugar, I get back on track with the 1-Day Refresh. It's such a great-tasting and simple way to lose weekend bloat and feel great again. I keep blends in my freezer for just such emergencies!"
—Carolyn K

I'm having a hard time staying off processed foods and diet sodas. Help!
Having them once in a while isn't the end of the world, but if you find it becoming a regular habit, then try doing the Reboot again. It will give your taste buds a hard reset from all that addicting sugar, salt, and fat.

NEED A 1-DAY REFRESH?

If you've had a weekend of pigging out or find processed foods sneaking back into your diet, get back on track by doing a one-day cleanse. Go back to Chapter 2, but make the entire batch of Base Blends—as if you were doing all three days. Then you'll have extra servings ready to go in your fridge, which will renew your habit of adding them to your everyday meals.

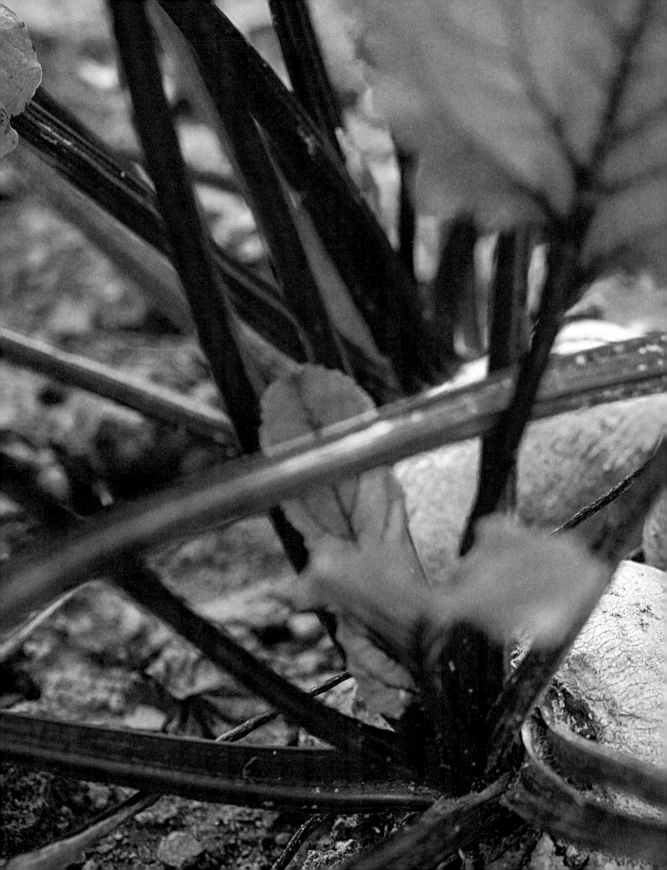

Part 2:
The Blends

Hungry for more? This section houses all the recipes for my fifteen nutrient-packed Base Blends—four of which you're already familiar with from the Reboot—and more than one hundred recipes for incredibly satisfying meals, snacks, desserts, and drinks you can make with them. They're game changers.

Each recipe in Chapters 4 and 5 has an icon designed to give you some at-a-glance info in case you have particular dietary requirements. Here's the key:

GF = Gluten free (there are 98 gluten-free recipes in this book!)

LC = Low carb (contains minimal carbohydrates—no more than 10 grams per serving)

V = Vegetarian (may include dairy, but no eggs, fish, poultry, or meat)

DF = Dairy free

Note: I don't call out those that are low-salt, low-sugar, low–saturated fat, or high-fiber because nearly every single recipe fits that bill.

Chapter 4:
Base Blends

EASY RECIPES FOR THE 15 COLORFUL BLENDS YOU'LL USE AGAIN AND AGAIN

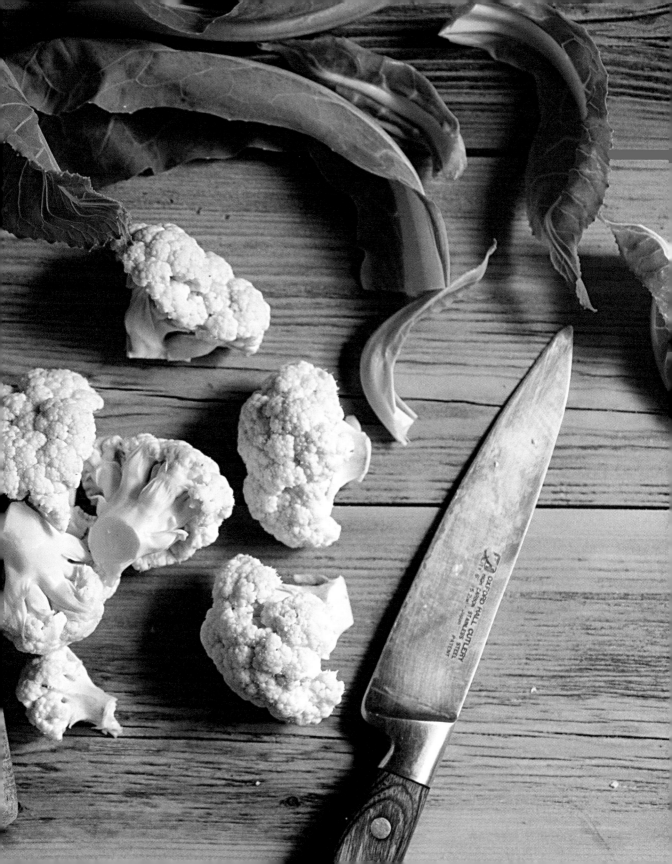

The Base Blends that follow are the foundation of every recipe in this book, and I've divided all fifteen of them into five color groups: white, orange, green, red, and purple, each with three variations. Most of the variations can be used interchangeably in the recipes you'll be making, so you can pick the blend in that color group that you like best, or play around with different ones. (There's a chart at the beginning of each recipe section that specifies which blends can be substituted for the one I call for.)

A couple of general tips: It's important to use a high-powered blender or food processor. (A regular blender won't work as well. It requires too much liquid to puree down.) When making more than one blend at a time, go from the lightest to darkest colors—for example, white, then orange, green, red, and purple. That way, you don't have to clean the blender in between batches. And remember to only add as much water as you need to puree the produce until smooth. The less you use, the better, for both consistency and concentrated nutrition. Start with almost no water and add it by the tablespoon just until the blend comes together. The amount you need will vary depending if you're using a high-powered blender—which requires almost no water—or a food processor. (For more blending tips, see page 14.) Finally, note that I call for tap water for steaming produce, but *filtered* water if it's an ingredient in a recipe that's going to be eaten.

"I'm not much of a gourmet cook, but these blends are so easy to make—just a few ingredients and a few minutes and you're done!" —Julie K.

I recommend having at least two Base Blends in your fridge or freezer at all times. Bang them out at once and you'll be good to go for days. The blends will keep for three days in the refrigerator, or three months in the freezer.

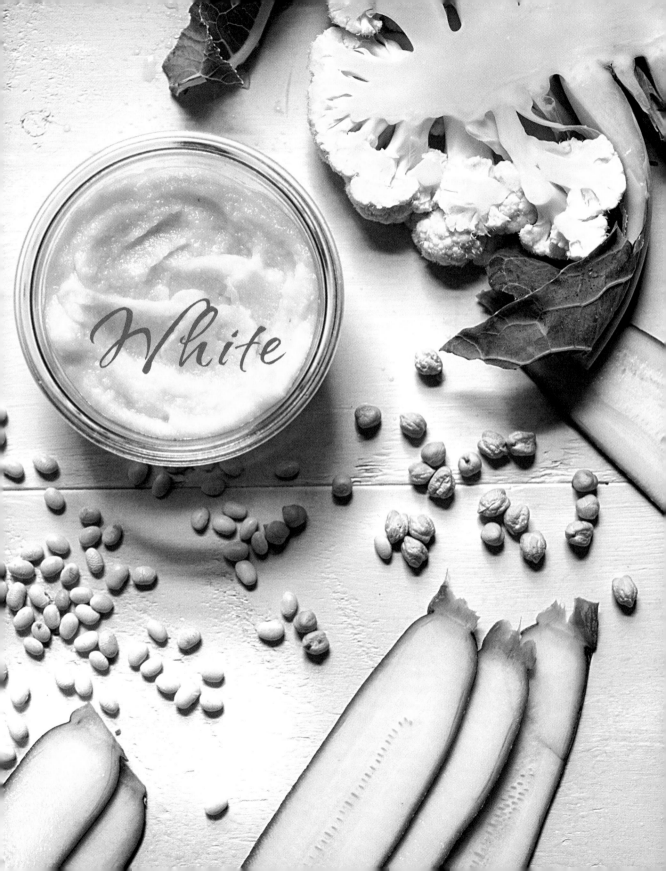

CHICKPEA-ZUCCHINI
BASE BLEND

• *Makes 2 ¹/₄ cups* •

Beans are amazing for you; some "blue zones" with the greatest longevity eat them as a dietary staple, but they can be calorically dense. So here I've added a mild-tasting vegetable that's super-low in calories to balance things out. If you prefer to use dried beans, soak them overnight and cook as directed.

1 15-ounce can chickpeas, drained and rinsed

2 medium zucchini, peeled and roughly chopped

Filtered water

Puree the beans and zucchini along with 3 to 4 tablespoons of filtered water until smooth, adding more water as necessary.

Nutrition facts (per ¹/₂ cup): 96 calories; 1 g fat; 218 mg sodium; 17 g carbs; 5 g fiber; 3 g sugar; 5 g protein

WHITE BEAN BASE BLEND

• Makes about 4 ¹/₂ cups •

GF
V
DF

Yes, I'm calling for a whole lotta beans here; but this is a puree that you'll use over and over, so you'll definitely go through this big batch because it is versatile: It can go savory and replace mayo or cream in a recipe, or go sweet and stand in for the butter or oil in baked goods. And it's so good you can even eat it straight up. Don't believe me? You'll find slight variations of this blend on tables all over Tuscany. And this freezes beautifully. If you'd rather not lug home so many cans, you can make this from dried beans. Just soak them overnight and cook according to the package directions.

4 15-ounce cans white beans,
   such as Great Northern,
   navy, butter, or cannellini,
   drained and rinsed

Filtered water

Puree the beans with ¼ to ⅓ cup filtered water and puree until smooth, adding more water as necessary.

Nutrition facts (per ¹/₂ cup): 156 calories; 2 g fat; 62 mg sodium; 26 g carbs; 8 g fiber; 1 g sugar; 9 g protein

CAULIFLOWER BASE BLEND

• *Makes 4 cups* •

GF
LC
V
DF

This is the lightest of all my blends; yet since it's a cruciferous vegetable, it has incredible health benefits. (See page 16.) Blending also makes it easier for your body to absorb cauliflower's beneficial phytonutrients. Win-win! Note: You can totally swap in frozen cauliflower florets here, if you'd like. Just run them under hot water to thaw them a little before putting them in your blender.

4 cups cauliflower florets (about 1 large, or 2 small heads)

Filtered water

Place a steamer basket into a large pot, pour in a few inches of tap water (make sure the water is below the bottom of the basket), and set it over high heat. Add the cauliflower and steam, covered, for 9 to 11 minutes, until fork-tender. Remove from the heat and puree the cooked cauliflower with ¼ cup of filtered water until smooth, adding more water as necessary.

Nutrition facts (per ¹/₂ cup): **21 calories; 0 g fat; 26 mg sodium; 5 g carbs; 2 g fiber; 2 g sugar; 2 g protein**

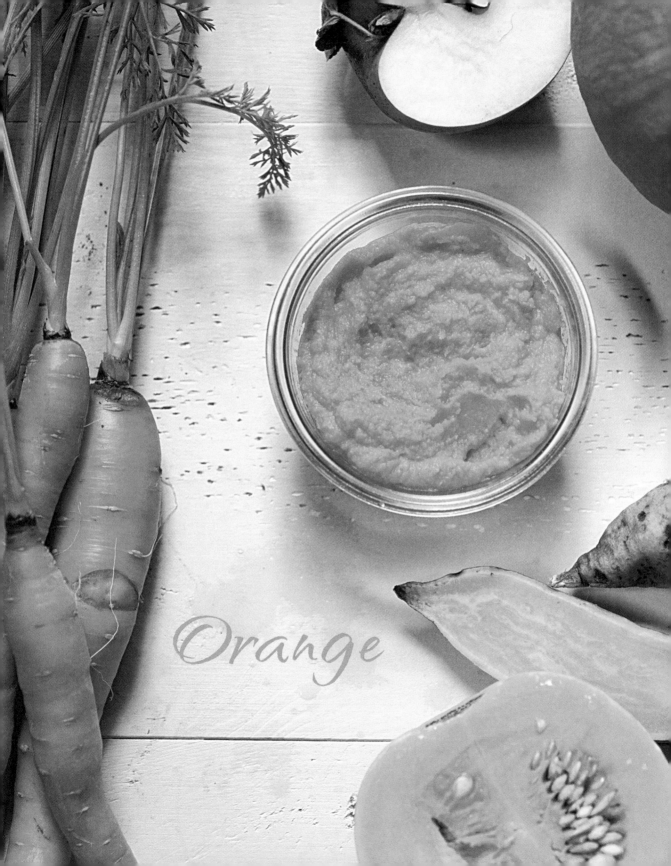

Orange

CARROT-SWEET POTATO BASE BLEND

• Makes 4 ¹/₂ cups •

This blend takes a bit more time than some of the others, but I have to tell you—it's my favorite child! It works in almost anything thanks to its creamy, deliciously sweet flavor profile. You can use it as a base for pasta sauce to take down the acidity, and it replaces cheese or butter in sweet and savory recipes. Don't drive yourself crazy dicing the veggies; a rough chop is fine. Just try to make them roughly the same size so they cook evenly. Some markets do sell frozen diced sweet potatoes. If you can find these timesavers, use them! Pick up some frozen carrots, too. Then you can skip the steaming and simply flash-thaw them by pouring hot water over both veggies and go directly to the blending step. You'll need about 4 cups of frozen chopped sweet potatoes and 3 cups of frozen chopped carrots total.

2 medium sweet potatoes or yams, peeled and roughly chopped

6 medium to large carrots, peeled and roughly chopped

Filtered water

Place a steamer basket into a large pot, pour in a few inches of tap water (make sure the water is below the bottom of the basket), and set it over high heat. Add the sweet potatoes and carrots and steam, covered, for 15 to 20 minutes, until fork-tender. Puree the veggies with 2 to 3 tablespoons of filtered water until smooth, adding more water as necessary.

Nutrition facts (per ¹/₂ cup): **47 calories; 1 g fat; 50 mg sodium; 11 g carbs; 2 g fiber; 4 g sugar; 1 g protein**

BUTTERNUT SQUASH-APPLE BASE BLEND

• Makes 2 ¹/₂ cups •

I lean on frozen squash to save time, but you can also buy the already peeled and diced kind you'll find in the produce section of most supermarkets and steam it for 15 minutes or so. If you have a little more time and want to deepen the flavor of the squash, prick a fresh butternut squash all over and bake it like a potato at 350 degrees for about 45 minutes, until soft. Allow it to cool slightly, then cut the squash in half lengthwise, remove the seeds, scoop out the flesh, and cube it. I discovered this method after almost cutting my hand off trying to slice into a wobbly, raw butternut squash. Never again!

1 ½ cups frozen diced butternut squash

2 medium apples, unpeeled, cored and roughly chopped

Filtered water

Place the squash in a large heatproof bowl and pour boiling water over it to thaw it; drain. Puree the squash and apples along with 2 to 3 tablespoons of filtered water until smooth, adding more water as necessary.

Nutrition facts (per ¹/₂ cup): **56 calories; 0 g fat; 1 mg sodium; 13 g carbs; 2 g fiber; 9 g sugar; 1 g protein**

PUMPKIN BASE BLEND

• *Makes 2 ²/₃ cups* •

GF
V
DF

If you can't find frozen pumpkin, pick up canned 100% pure pumpkin—not the sugary pie filling kind. It's a huge timesaver and nearly as nutritious as the frozen stuff. I use it all year long. If you're feeling ambitious and want to roast your own, halve and seed a small pumpkin, place it on a baking sheet, and pop it in a 350-degree oven for 40 to 50 minutes (depending on the size of the pumpkin), until it cuts easily with a knife. Just look for good eating types, like sugar pumpkins or baby bears; you don't want to wrestle the jack-o'-lantern kind, nor would it taste very good.

4 cups diced frozen pumpkin

Filtered water

Place the pumpkin in a large heatproof bowl and pour boiling water over it to thaw it; drain. Puree the pumpkin along with 2 to 3 tablespoons of filtered water until smooth, adding more water as necessary.

Nutrition facts (per ¹/₂ cup): **75 calories; 0 g fat; 0 mg sodium; 15 g carbs; 6 g fiber; 6 g sugar; 2 g protein**

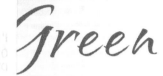
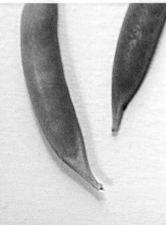

BROCCOLI-PEA-SPINACH BASE BLEND

• *Makes 4 cups* •

In many cases, I prefer the ease of frozen fruits and veggies, but go for the fresh, prewashed, bagged baby spinach here—it has a milder flavor. If you must use frozen (the chopped spinach that comes in a block), only use 1 cup for this recipe. Oh, and if you like fresh baby kale better than spinach, go ahead and swap it in.

4 cups broccoli florets, fresh or frozen

3 cups frozen sweet green peas

4 cups baby spinach

Filtered water

Place a steamer basket into a large pot, pour in a few inches of tap water (make sure the water is below the bottom of the basket), and set it over high heat. Add the broccoli and steam, covered, for about 10 minutes if fresh, or about 2 minutes if frozen, until just tender. Add the frozen peas to the basket for the last 2 minutes of steaming. Pulse the spinach in a high-powered blender a few times to reduce its volume. Add the steamed veggies along with 2 to 3 tablespoons of filtered water, and puree until smooth, adding more water as necessary.

Nutrition facts (per ¹/₂ cup): 42 calories; 0 g fat; 67 mg sodium; 7 g carbs; 2 g fiber; 2 g sugar; 3 g protein

SWEET PEA–BABY KALE
BASE BLEND

• Makes about 3 cups •

As with baby spinach, I like to use fresh baby kale for this blend because of its milder flavor. But if you're into frozen, then only use 2 cups of the chopped stuff you buy in a block.

3 cups sweet green frozen peas

8 cups loosely packed baby kale

Filtered water

Place the peas in a large heatproof bowl. Bring a medium pot of tap water to a boil, then pour the water over the peas to thaw them. Meanwhile, put the kale into a high-powered blender and pulse a few times to reduce its volume. Drain the peas and add them to the blender, along with 3 to 4 tablespoons of filtered water, and puree until smooth, adding more water as necessary.

Nutrition facts (per $^1/_2$ cup) : 83 calories; 0 g fat; 175 mg sodium; 15 g carbs; 4 g fiber; 3 g sugar; 6 g protein

GF
V
DF

SWEET PEA BASE BLEND

• Makes 2 ¹/₂ cups •

Be sure to look for sweet baby peas—they're much more delicious than bigger, starchier regular peas. And yes, go frozen. Can you imagine shelling that many fresh peas? Yikes!

4 cups sweet green frozen peas

Filtered water

Place the peas in a large heatproof bowl. Bring a medium pot of tap water to a boil, then pour the water over the peas to thaw them. Drain, then blend the peas with ¼ cup filtered water and puree until smooth, adding more water as necessary.

Nutrition facts (per ¹/₂ cup): **85 calories; 0 g fat; 242 mg sodium; 14 g carbs; 5 g fiber; 5 g sugar; 6 g protein**

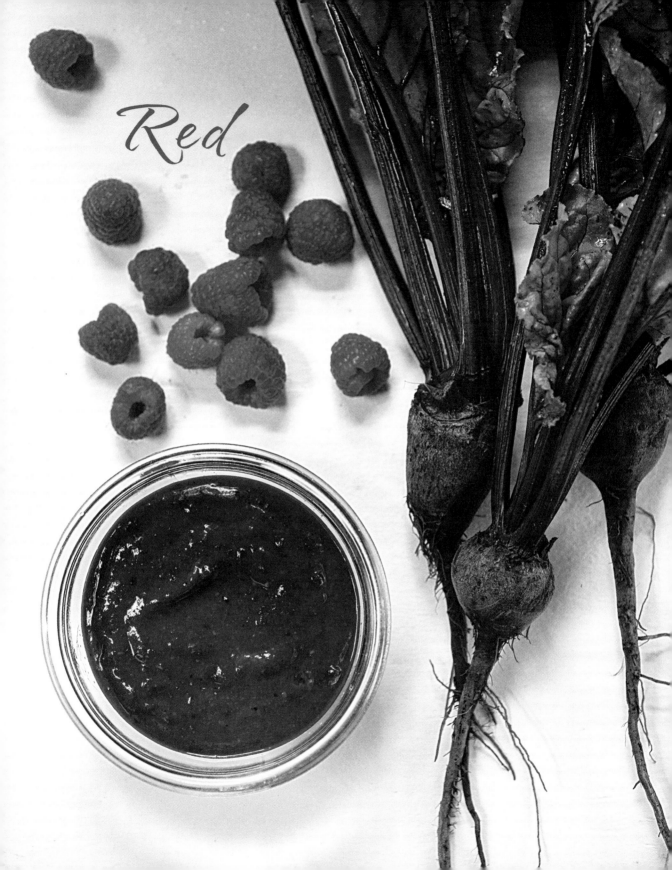

Red

RASPBERRY-BEET BASE BLEND

• Makes 2 ³/₄ cups •

This blend is the most gorgeous color—and that rich pigment is where its great nutrition comes from. And even if you think you don't like beets, you've got to give this a try. The raspberries take down some of the earthiness of the veggie; but because both have lots of natural sugars, you can sweeten many dishes with this blend without adding actual sweeteners (or at least use much less of them). I love to roast beets to enhance those natural sugars, but if you don't have time, it's fine to sub in canned peeled-and-cooked beets, or the ready-to-eat kind you can find in the fridge case in the produce aisle.

2 medium beets

4 cups frozen raspberries

Filtered water

Preheat the oven to 400 degrees. Cut the ends off the beets, peel, and cut them into chunks (around 1 inch). Place on a baking sheet and roast for about 35 minutes, until tender. Meanwhile, rinse the raspberries in cold water to thaw slightly; drain well. Puree the berries and beets with 2 to 3 tablespoons of filtered water until smooth, adding more water as necessary.

Nutrition facts (per ¹/₂ cup): 49 calories; 0 g fat; 23 mg sodium; 17 g carbs; 7 g fiber; 11 g sugar; 1 g protein

RASPBERRY BASE BLEND

• Makes 2 cups •

Raspberries are super-high in fiber—8 grams worth in just 1 cup—and this berries-only blend is so fresh and the perfect balance of sweet and tart. Your blend will still have some seeds, but just go with it; once it's incorporated into recipes you won't notice them.

4 cups frozen raspberries

Filtered water

Rinse the raspberries in cold water to thaw slightly; drain well. Puree the berries with 2 to 3 tablespoons of filtered water until smooth, adding more water as necessary.

Nutrition facts (per ½ cup): **50 calories; 0 g fat; 0 mg sodium; 20 g carbs; 8 g fiber; 12 g sugar; 1 g protein**

BEET BASE BLEND

• Makes ³/₄ cup •

Lately, athletes have been going bonkers for beets, consuming them to increase blood and oxygen flow and improve their performance. And chefs have, too: Beets are popping up on the menus of ultra-chic restaurants these days. So worth trying! If you don't want to go to the trouble of roasting the beets yourself, you can use a 14.5-ounce can of ready-to-eat beets (drained) in place of the fresh ones called for below, or use the precooked kind you'll find in the produce section of many grocery stores.

2 medium beets

Filtered water

Preheat the oven to 400 degrees. Cut the ends off the beets, peel, and cut them into chunks. Place on a baking sheet and roast for about 35 minutes, until tender. Puree the beets with 1 to 2 tablespoons filtered water until smooth, adding more water as necessary.

Nutrition facts (per ¹/₂ cup): **47 calories; 0 g fat; 85 mg sodium; 11 g carbs; 3 g fiber; 7 g sugar; 2 g protein**

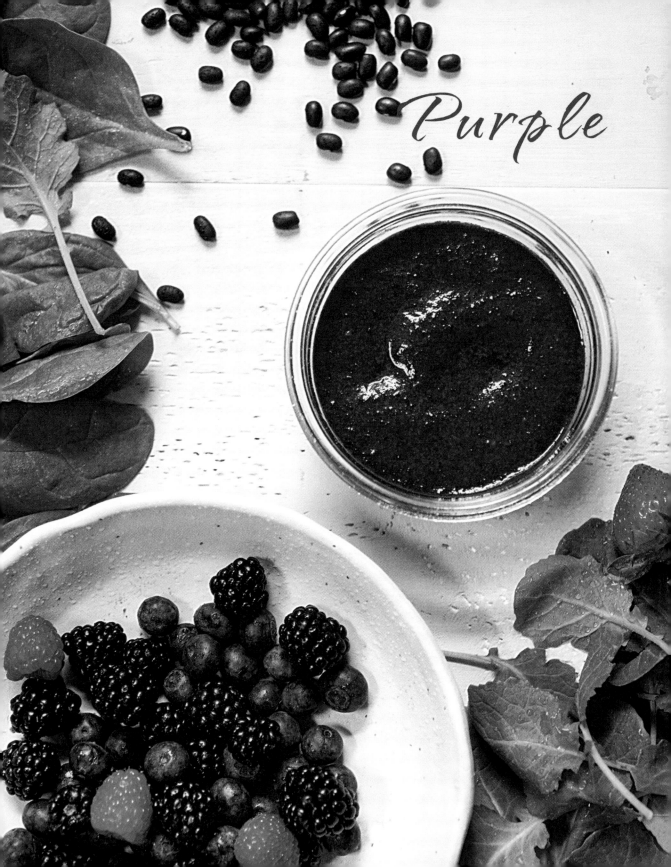

Purple

BLUEBERRY-BABY SPINACH BASE BLEND

• *Makes 2 cups* •

I know: Blueberries and spinach are two things that don't sound like they'd go together. But they actually complement each other beautifully somehow. The berries give the spinach a slightly sweet taste that's still mild enough to marry well with almost any dish, whether sweet or savory. There's a lot of spinach here, so I'd recommend using the bagged kind that's already washed and ready to go.

6 cups baby spinach

3 cups frozen blueberries, ideally wild

Filtered water

Place the spinach into a high-powered blender and pulse a few times to reduce its volume. Give the blueberries a quick rinse in cold water just to thaw them slightly and add them to the blender along with 1 to 2 tablespoons of filtered water and puree until smooth.

Nutrition facts (per ¹/₂ cup): **74 calories; 0 g fat; 54 mg sodium; 16 g carbs; 5 g fiber; 10 g sugar; 2 g protein**

MIXED BERRY–BABY KALE BASE BLEND

• *Makes 2 cups* •

I usually use frozen berries, especially if they're not in season. They're cheaper than fresh, tend to have more antioxidants, and are easier to blend. Don't worry about buying multiple bags and mixing them together; you can find bags of assorted berries already mixed in the freezer case. Note: This recipe calls for fresh baby kale, which I prefer, but if you have to use frozen, drop the amount called for to 1 ½ cups.

6 cups baby kale, washed

4 cups frozen mixed berries

Filtered water

Place the kale in a high-powered blender and pulse a few times to reduce its volume. Give the berries a quick rinse in cold water just to thaw them slightly and add them to the blender along with 1 to 2 tablespoons of filtered water and puree until smooth.

Nutrition facts (per ¹/₂ cup): 104 calories; 0 g fat; 26 mg sodium; 24 g carbs; 7 g fiber; 11 g sugar; 13 g protein

BLACK BEAN–BLUEBERRY–BABY KALE BASE BLEND

• Makes 4 cups •

I keep several BPA-free cans of beans on hand at all times, since they last so long. But if you're a dried bean kind of person, feel free to sub them in (they'll need to be soaked overnight and cooked, of course). And if you're not a lover of kale, go ahead and swap in fresh baby spinach or your favorite leafy green. I'm all about options!

4 cups baby kale

2 cups frozen blueberries, ideally wild

2 15-ounce cans black beans, drained and rinsed

Filtered water

Place the kale into a high-powered blender and pulse a few times. Rinse the blueberries in cold water to thaw them slightly. Add the berries and the beans to the blender along with 1 to 2 tablespoons of filtered water and puree until smooth, adding more water as necessary.

Nutrition facts (per ¹/₂ cup): **121 calories; 1 g fat; 16 mg sodium; 23 g carbs; 7 g fiber; 3 g sugar; 7 g protein**

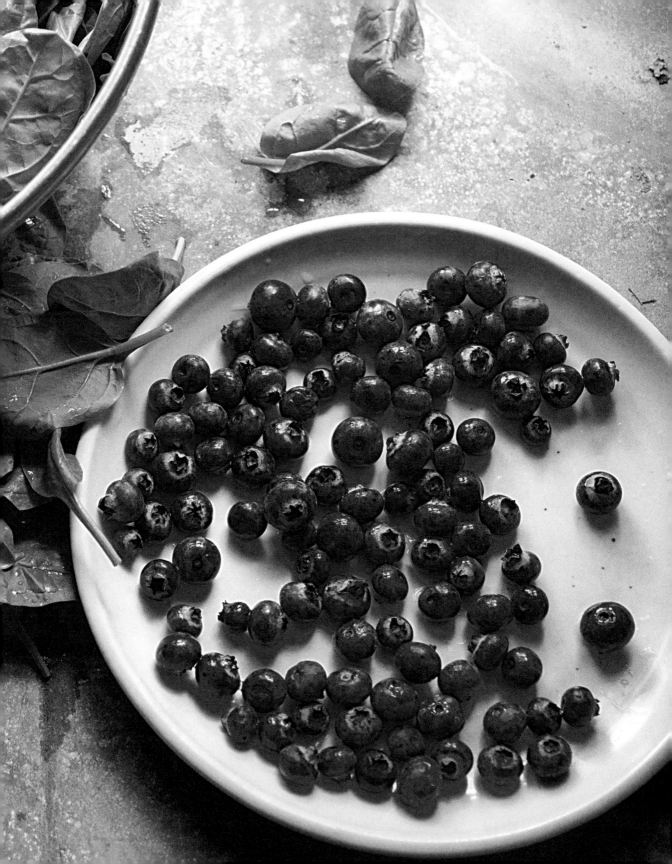

Chapter 5

Blends Recipes

DELICIOUS MEALS, SNACKS, AND—YES—DESSERTS THAT INCORPORATE BLENDS TO UP THE NUTRITION AND SKINNY FACTOR

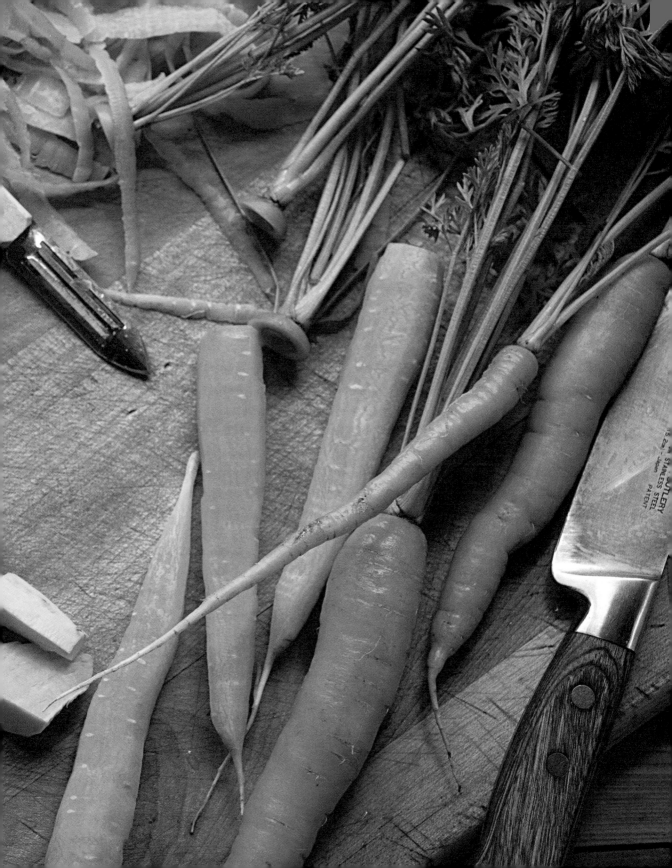

This section is where you get to use your Base Blends as a tool to magically change the way you cook. All of the recipes in this chapter were designed with one thing in mind: giving you the delicious comfort foods you crave in a healthier, lightened-up way—with all the taste and satisfaction. And they just make you feel good. I love to eat, and I love good food. And I believe that life's too short to eat like a rabbit just so you can fit into a particular jeans size. These recipes mean you don't have to. You don't have to give up on taste, richness, or portion size; my blends invisibly transform every dish into a better version of itself. They are a way to literally have your chocolate cake and eat it, too. Enjoy!

Wake

Satisfying A.M. Meals and Superfast,
Out-the-Door Solutions

Below you'll find a list of all the breakfast recipes, along with the blends they call for. Use it as a key to figuring out what to make based on the blends you have on hand. In many cases, you can also use another blend in place of the one that's called for in the recipe, to give you even more versatility. Mornings just got that much easier!

THE DISH	THE BASE BLEND
Creamy Berry Blend	Blueberry–Baby Spinach Base Blend (or Mixed Berry–Baby Kale Base Blend)
Cinnamon–Sweet Potato Blend	Carrot–Sweet Potato Base Blend (or any Orange Base Blend)
Avo-Berry Blend	Raspberry Base Blend (or Raspberry-Beet Base Blend)
Chocolate Crepes	Blueberry–Baby Spinach Base Blend (or Mixed Berry–Baby Kale Base Blend)
Sweet Potato Crepes	Carrot–Sweet Potato Base Blend (or any Orange Base Blend)
"No More Muffin Top!" Blueberry Muffin Tops	Chickpea-Zucchini Base Blend (or any Orange Base Blend)
Skinny Sweet Potato Donut Bites	Carrot–Sweet Potato Base Blend (or any Orange Base Blend)
Broccoli-Cheddar Mini Frittata	Broccoli-Pea-Spinach Base Blend (or any Green Base Blend)
Berry Crunchy Smoothie Bowl	Raspberry-Beet Base Blend (or Raspberry Base Blend)
Chai Tea Smoothie Bowl	Butternut Squash–Apple Base Blend (or any Orange Base Blend)
Banana-Chia To-Go Cup	Carrot–Sweet Potato Base Blend (or any Orange Base Blend)
Blueberry-Chia To-Go Cup	Blueberry–Baby Spinach Base Blend
Cinnamon-Oat Protein Pancakes	Carrot–Sweet Potato Base Blend (or any Orange Base Blend)
Cocoa Protein Pancakes	Blueberry–Baby Spinach Base Blend (or Mixed Berry–Baby Kale Base Blend)
Berry Detox Shake	Blueberry–Baby Spinach Base Blend (or Mixed Berry–Baby Kale Base Blend)

THE DISH	THE BASE BLEND
DIY Cream Cheese	Raspberry Base Blend
Warm Butternut Squash–Apple Breakfast Soup	Butternut Squash–Apple Base Blend (or any Orange Base Blend)
Cheesy Kale-Basil Soufflé	Sweet Pea–Baby Kale Base Blend (or any Green Base Blend)
Lemon-Chia Quick Bread	Butternut Squash–Apple Base Blend (or any Orange Base Blend)

1-MINUTE MEALS

Yes, they're really that fast. These speedy breakfasts are Base Blends that have a few little extras thrown in just to punch up the flavor. In these recipes, the blends are the total stars. They give you more flexibility and allow you to fix something in seconds—from a blend you already have on hand—rather than make a more involved recipe.

CREAMY BERRY BLEND

GF
V

• Makes 1 serving •

1 cup **Blueberry–Baby Spinach Base Blend** (page 98)

2 tablespoons plain low-fat Greek yogurt

1 teaspoon raw honey

3 to 4 ice cubes

Low-fat milk or unsweetened plant-based milk

Place the first 4 ingredients into a high-powered blender, add a splash of milk to thin the mixture, and puree until smooth, adding a bit more milk, as needed.

Nutrition facts: 189 calories; 0 g fat; 122 mg sodium; 40 g carbs; 9 g fiber; 27 g sugar; 7 g protein

CINNAMON–SWEET POTATO BLEND

• Makes 1 serving •

1 cup **Carrot–Sweet Potato Base Blend**
(page 86)

½ tablespoon extra-virgin olive oil

2 tablespoons low-fat milk or unsweetened

plant-based milk

½ tablespoon pure maple syrup

Pinch of ground cinnamon

Pinch of sea salt

Warm all of the ingredients in a small saucepan over medium-low heat, mixing well to combine, and serve.

Nutrition facts: 194 calories; 8 g fat; 115 mg sodium; 30 g carbs; 5 g fiber; 15 g sugar; **3 g protein**

* *(if using plant-based milk)*

AVO-BERRY BLEND

• Makes 1 serving •

¾ cup **Raspberry Base Blend** (page 95)

¼ avocado

2 tablespoons plain low-fat Greek yogurt

½ tablespoon raw honey

3 to 4 ice cubes

Low-fat milk or unsweetened plant-based milk

Place the first 5 ingredients into a high-powered blender, add a splash of milk to thin the mixture, and puree until smooth, adding a bit more milk, as needed.

Nutrition facts: 184 calories; 5 g fat; 17 mg sodium; 43 g carbs; 14 g fiber; 28 g sugar; **6 g protein**

CHOCOLATE CREPES

Makes 4 servings • Serving size: 2 crepes

People think crepes are so hard to make, but they're just like making pancakes with a thinner batter. To make them easier to flip, run a spatula around the edges of the crepe to loosen it, then (carefully!) grab one side with your fingers and quickly flip it over. Keep in mind that while the batter makes enough for 4 servings of crepes, the fillings below are for a single portion—so increase the quantities if you're sharing.

1 cup liquid egg whites

½ cup low-fat milk (or unsweetened plant-based milk)

2 teaspoons pure vanilla extract

⅛ teaspoon sea salt

½ cup whole grain pastry flour

½ cup **Blueberry–Baby Spinach Base Blend** (page 98)

2 packets stevia (1 teaspoon total)

2 dashes ground cinnamon

1 tablespoon unsweetened cocoa powder, plus more for dusting

Nonstick cooking spray

Filling option 1 (for 2 crepes):
2 tablespoons part-skim ricotta cheese

¼ cup fresh berries

½ tablespoon raw honey

Filling option 2 (for 2 crepes):
2 tablespoons plain low-fat Greek yogurt

½ medium banana, sliced

½ tablespoon raw honey

In a large bowl, whisk together all ingredients for the crepe batter until completely smooth. Mist a small (about 8-inch) nonstick frying pan with cooking spray and set over medium-high heat. (Be sure to generously coat the bottom and sides.) Pour ¼ cup of batter into the hot pan and swirl it so it evenly covers the bottom of the pan. Cook the crepe for about 1 minute, until the top is no longer wet and the edges start to brown. Loosen the edges with a spatula, flip, and cook the other side for another minute. Put your choice of filling into the center of the crepe and allow to melt for 1 minute, then fold the crepe into quarters. Remove to a plate and dust with cocoa powder. Repeat with the remaining batter, re-spraying the pan before making each crepe.

Nutrition facts (per serving for filling #1): 210 calories; 4 g fat; 273 mg sodium; 33 g carbs; 4 g fiber; 15 g sugar; 12 g protein

Nutrition facts (per serving for filling #2): 214 calories; 1 g fat; 207 mg sodium; 41 g carbs; 4 g fiber; 20 g sugar; 12 g protein

SWEET POTATO CREPES

Makes 4 servings • Serving size: 2 crepes

These ridiculously-easy-to-make crepes can be filled with either savory or sweet ingredients. Note that the batter makes enough for 4 servings of crepes, but the fillings listed are for just 1 serving—so up the amount accordingly, if needed. Stack any extra crepes between sheets of waxed paper, wrap in plastic, and store in the fridge for 3 days—or freeze them for up to 3 months. Just thaw them before using by warming them in a skillet before adding your filling of choice.

1 cup liquid egg whites

½ cup low-fat milk (or unsweetened plant-based milk)

2 teaspoons pure vanilla extract

⅛ teaspoon sea salt

½ cup whole grain pastry flour

½ cup **Carrot–Sweet Potato Base Blend** (page 86)

2 packets stevia (1 teaspoon total)

¼ teaspoon ground cinnamon

Nonstick cooking spray

Filling option 1 (for 2 crepes):
2 tablespoons shredded Gruyère cheese

2 thin slices no-nitrates-added ham

Filling option 2 (for 2 crepes):
1 tablespoon almond butter

½ medium banana, sliced

In a large bowl, whisk together all ingredients for the crepe batter until completely smooth. Mist a small (about 8-inch) nonstick frying pan with cooking spray and set over medium-high heat. (Be sure to generously coat the bottom and sides.) Pour ¼ cup of the batter onto the hot pan and swirl it so it evenly covers the bottom of the pan. Cook the crepe for about 1 minute, until the top is no longer wet and the edges start to brown. Loosen the edges with a spatula, flip, and cook the other side for another minute. Put your choice of filling into the center of the crepe and allow to melt for 1 minute, then fold the crepe into quarters. Repeat with the remaining batter, re-spraying the pan before making each crepe.

Nutrition facts (per serving for filling #1): **194** calories; 6 g fat; 434 mg sodium; 17 g carbs; 2 g fiber; 3 g sugar; 17 g protein

Nutrition facts (per serving for filling #2): **259** calories; 8 g fat; 247 mg sodium; 35 g carbs; 4 g fiber; 12 g sugar; 10 g protein

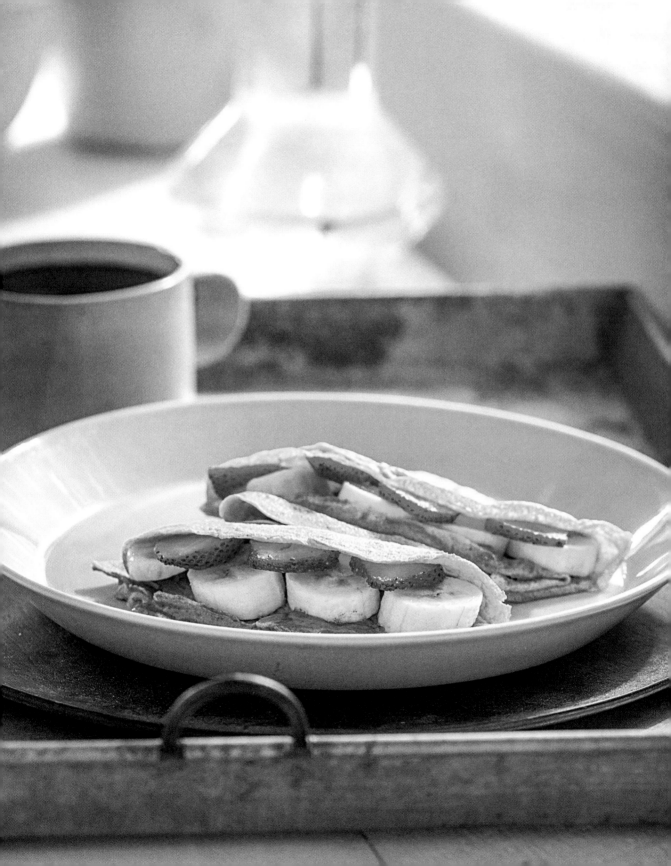

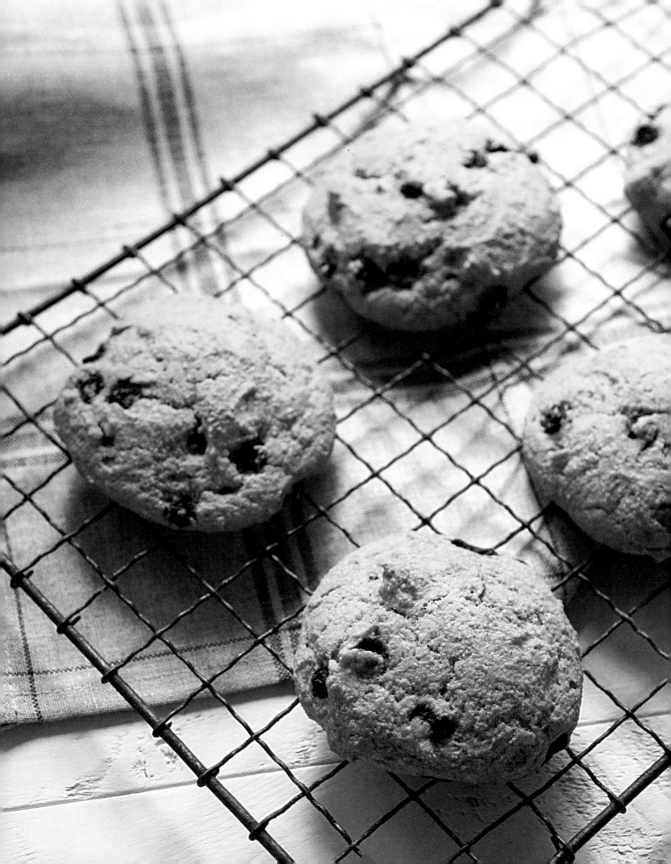

"NO MORE MUFFIN TOP!" BLUEBERRY MUFFIN TOPS

DF

Makes 8 servings • Serving size: 1 muffin top

It's the part of the muffin you most want to eat anyway, am I right? These give you the same crisp-around-the-edges and cakey center, but they're made easily on a baking sheet, and the nutritious blend stands in for much of the fat you'd normally use in a muffin recipe, which slashes the calories significantly. I defy you to say the same about your low-fat Starbucks muffin.

3 tablespoons canola or light olive oil

1 large egg

¾ cup **Chickpea-Zucchini Base Blend** (page 82)

1 teaspoon pure vanilla extract

6 tablespoons raw honey

1 ¼ cups whole grain pastry flour

1 teaspoon baking powder

½ teaspoon baking soda

½ teaspoon sea salt

¾ cup wild blueberries, fresh or frozen

Preheat the oven to 350 degrees. In a large bowl, stir together all ingredients until smooth. Line a baking sheet with parchment paper and place ¼-cup scoops of batter onto the baking sheet, leaving 2 inches of space between each one. Bake for 16 to 18 minutes, until the edges are golden brown.

Nutrition facts (per serving): 181 calories; 6 g fat; 335 mg sodium; 29 g carbs; 3 g fiber; 12 g sugar; 4 g protein

SKINNY SWEET POTATO DONUT BITES

Makes 6 servings • Serving size: 4 donut bites (or 2 mini muffin bites)

One summer, I visited Portland, Maine, where they're famous for potato donuts—which are great, but weigh about 2 pounds each! I came home inspired to make them, only *waaay* lighter and healthier. Mine use sweet potatoes and carrots and I bake them instead of frying them. OMG are they delish.

For the donuts

Nonstick cooking spray

½ cup plus 2 tablespoons whole grain pastry flour

¼ teaspoon ground cinnamon

¼ teaspoon sea salt

1 teaspoon baking powder

¼ cup canola or light olive oil

¼ cup pure maple syrup

1 large egg

2 tablespoons plain low-fat Greek yogurt

½ cup **Carrot–Sweet Potato Base Blend** (page 86)

½ teaspoon pure vanilla extract

For dusting the tops

1 tablespoon organic sugar (optional)

½ teaspoon cinnamon

Pinch of sea salt

Preheat the oven to 350 degrees. Generously mist a mini donut or mini muffin tin with cooking spray. In a large bowl, combine the flour, cinnamon, salt, and baking powder. In a medium bowl, whisk together the oil, maple syrup, egg, yogurt, the blend, and the vanilla. Stir the dry mixture into the wet ingredients until just combined. Spoon the batter into the baking tin, filling each individual well about three-quarters full. Bake for 16 minutes, until a toothpick comes out clean. To dust the tops: Mix the sugar (if using), cinnamon, and salt in a small bowl. Allow the donuts to cool or dive in while they're warm. Lightly mist the tops of the donuts with cooking spray and dust with the sugar mixture.

Nutrition facts (per serving): 191 calories; 11 g fat; 385 mg sodium; 22 g carbs; 2 g fiber; 11 g sugar; 3 g protein

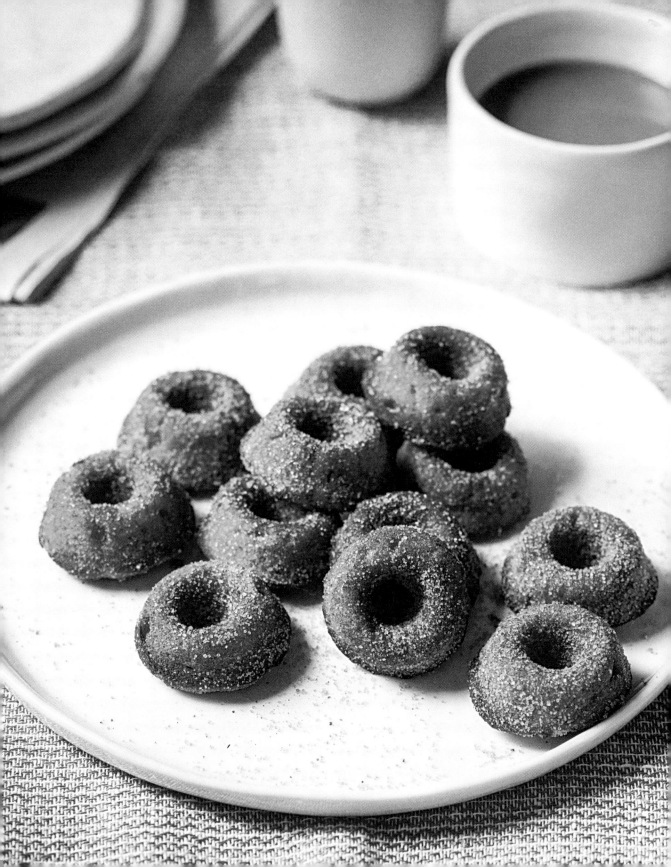

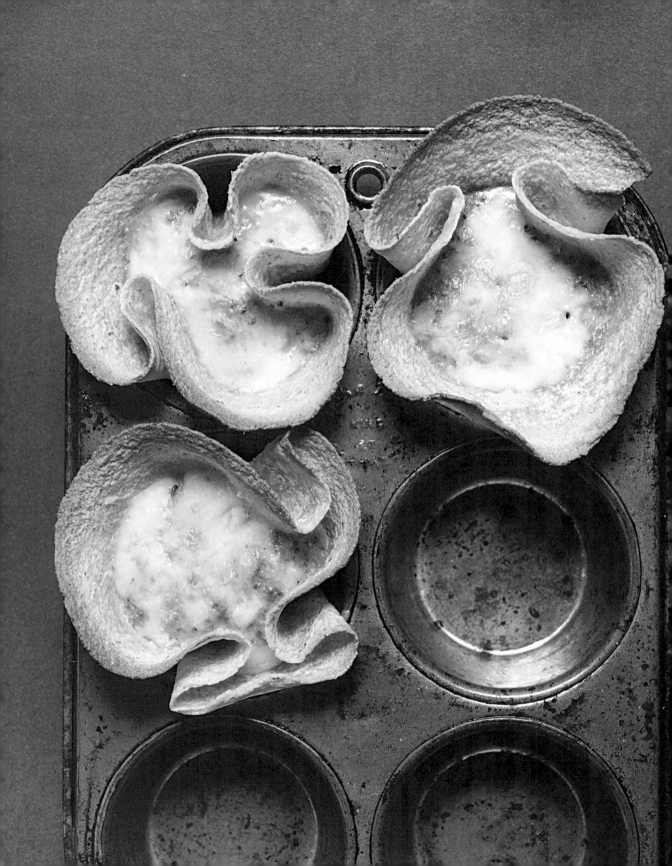

BROCCOLI-CHEDDAR
MINI FRITTATA

Makes 6 servings • Serving size: 1 frittata

In the morning, it's easy for a healthy breakfast to go out the window. So I make these ahead when I'm not in a rush, and then pop one in the toaster oven to warm before jetting out the door. They freeze perfectly, too. You can make these minus the tortilla, but I like that it gives this meal real portability.

Nonstick cooking spray

6 6-inch corn tortillas

4 large eggs

1 tablespoon chia seeds

⅔ cup shredded sharp cheddar cheese, divided

¼ teaspoon sea salt

½ cup **Broccoli-Pea-Spinach Base Blend** (page 90)

¾ cup finely chopped raw broccoli florets

Preheat the oven to 375 degrees. Mist a muffin tin with nonstick cooking spray. Wrap tortillas in a damp paper towel and microwave for 30 seconds to make them pliable. Gently press 1 into each of 6 muffin cups. In a large bowl, whisk together the eggs, chia seeds, ¼ cup of the cheese, salt, the blend, and the broccoli. Pour ¼ cup of the egg mixture into each muffin cup and top with the remaining cheese. Bake for 22 minutes, until the eggs are just set. Serve warm. Leftover frittatas freeze well for up to 3 months.

Nutrition facts (per serving): 162 calories; 8 g fat; 258 mg sodium; 12 g carbs; 3 g fiber; 1 g sugar; 10 g protein

BERRY CRUNCHY SMOOTHIE BOWL

Makes 2 servings • Serving size: $^2/_3$ cup smoothie, plus toppings

If you've never heard of smoothie bowls, they're basically a thicker version of the kind you'd serve in a glass and sip through a straw. Then you add toppings for texture and a nutritional boost. Here, the strong, lovable flavor of raspberries mellows out the beets—and gives you an incredible dose of phytonutrients. Don't skip the topping at the end; it gives the dish great crunch and makes it feel substantial.

¾ cup **Raspberry-Beet Base Blend** (page 94)

½ cup no-sugar-added pomegranate juice (or freshly squeezed orange juice)

2 teaspoons raw honey

1 cup plain low-fat Greek yogurt

½ cup frozen blueberries

3 teaspoons chia seeds, divided

3 tablespoons rolled oats (gluten free)

1 tablespoon slivered unsalted almonds

Pinch of ground cinnamon

Puree the blend, juice, honey, yogurt, blueberries, and 2 teaspoons of the chia seeds until smooth. In a small bowl combine the oats, almonds, cinnamon, and the remaining teaspoon of chia seeds. Pour the smoothie into 2 bowls, top each with half of the oat mixture, and serve.

Nutrition facts (per serving): **224 calories; 6 g fat; 31 mg sodium; 42 g carbs; 10 g fiber; 25 g sugar; 7 g protein**

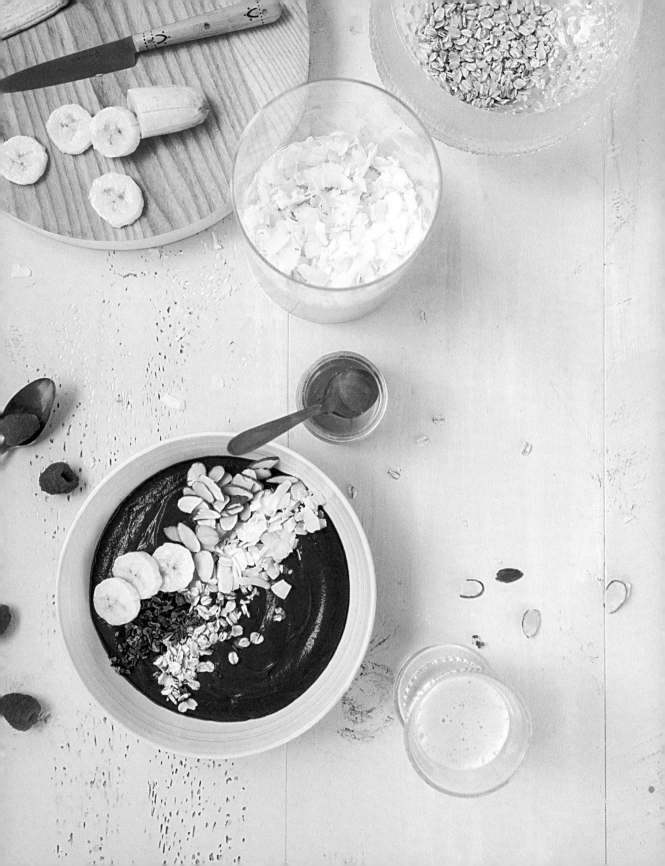

CHAI TEA SMOOTHIE BOWL

Makes 2 servings • Serving size: ²/₃ cup smoothie, plus toppings

I'm a big tea drinker and I love the mix of exotic spices—cinnamon, cardamom, ginger—in chai tea. It also gives you a gentle boost of caffeine so you could even skip your morning joe! I like to make several batches (without the toppings) and freeze in individual servings. Then all you have to do is thaw it in the fridge overnight, mix it up, and done! You've got breakfast in less than a minute.

2 chai tea bags, steeped for 3 to 4 minutes in 1 cup boiling water

1 cup unsweetened almond milk (or any milk or plant-based milk)

1 to 2 teaspoons raw honey

1 frozen banana*

½ cup **Butternut Squash–Apple Base Blend** (page 87)

Ground cinnamon

3 tablespoons rolled oats (gluten free)

1 tablespoon slivered unsalted almonds

1 teaspoon chia seeds or ground flaxseed

2 tablespoons plain low-fat Greek yogurt

After the tea has steeped, toss the tea bags and allow the tea to cool for 1 minute. Puree the tea, almond milk, honey, banana, the blend, and a dash of cinnamon until smooth. In a small bowl combine the oats, almonds, chia seeds or flaxseed, and a pinch of cinnamon. Pour the smoothie into 2 bowls, top each with half of the oat mixture and 1 tablespoon Greek yogurt, and serve.

* Peel and roughly chop ripe bananas and store them in individual freezer bags.

Nutrition facts (per serving): 194 calories; 6 g fat; 96 mg sodium; 33 g carbs; 5 g fiber; 17 g sugar; 5 g protein

BANANA-CHIA TO-GO CUP

6F
V

• *Makes 1 serving* •

This recipe was inspired by the amazing banana pudding at Magnolia Bakery in New York City. They're famous for it—and for good reason. It's to-die-for delicious! But it also contains an unspeakable amount of cream, sugar, and other unhealthy ingredients. So I made a slimmed-down version that you can have for breakfast. Best of all: It's totally portable. Take a couple of minutes to assemble it the night before, which will allow the chia seeds to set up into a thick, pudding-like consistency. In the morning, all you have to do is add a dollop of Greek yogurt and get out there.

2 tablespoons chia seeds
  (preferably white chia)

¼ cup water

¼ cup unsweetened coconut
  or almond milk

¼ cup **Carrot–Sweet Potato
  Base Blend** (page 86)

½ banana, mashed

Pinch of sea salt

Pinch of ground cinnamon

1 tablespoon plain low-fat
  Greek yogurt

In a travel mug, stir together the chia, water, coconut milk, the blend, the banana, salt, and cinnamon until combined. Cover and place in the refrigerator overnight to set. (The mixture starts out as a liquid, but will firm up by morning.) In the A.M., top the pudding with the Greek yogurt and off you go!

{ *Nutrition facts (per serving)*: **237** calories; **11 g** fat; **80 mg** sodium; **32 g** carbs; **13 g** fiber; **10 g** sugar; **9 g** protein }

BLUEBERRY-CHIA TO-GO CUP

• Makes 1 serving •

The chia seeds in this easy recipe transform it into an amazingly thick, custardy consistency overnight—with a little bit of chew that reminds me of the tapioca pudding I used to love as a kid. Don't be thrown by the fact that you have to assemble this ahead. It takes literally two minutes.

2 tablespoons chia seeds (preferably white chia)

¼ cup unsweetened coconut or almond milk

½ cup **Blueberry–Baby Spinach Base Blend** (page 98)

½ tablespoon raw honey or pure maple syrup

1 tablespoon plain low-fat Greek yogurt

In a travel mug, stir together the chia, coconut milk, the blend, and the honey until combined. Cover and place in the refrigerator overnight to set. (The mixture will look very liquid but will firm up by morning.) In the A.M., top the pudding with the Greek yogurt and go.

Nutrition facts (per serving): 266 calories; 11 g fat; 108 mg sodium; 38 g carbs; 15 g fiber; 19 g sugar; 10 g protein

CINNAMON-OAT PROTEIN PANCAKES

Makes 14 pancakes • Serving size: 6 pancakes

Pancakes are almost always just carbs, carbs, carbs—simple carbs. They're hunger bombs that make you more ravenous than if you'd eaten nothing. So I came up with a version that's more nutritious and just as satisfying. I also added muscle-building protein: A serving of these has as much protein as 2 ½ large eggs! Leftovers freeze really well, too. Just pop them in the toaster to reheat.

2 tablespoons part-skim ricotta cheese

1 large egg

¼ teaspoon sea salt

¼ teaspoon ground cinnamon

1 teaspoon pure vanilla extract

¼ cup **Carrot–Sweet Potato Base Blend** (page 86)

¼ cup low-fat milk (or unsweetened plant-based milk)

1 tablespoon pure maple syrup

½ cup plus 1 tablespoon rolled oats, finely ground (gluten free)

2 scoops unsweetened plain or vanilla protein powder

Nonstick cooking spray

In a large bowl, whisk together all of the ingredients. Mist a griddle or large skillet with cooking spray and set over medium heat. Pour rounded tablespoons of batter into the pan and cook until bubbles begin to set around the edges and the pancakes are golden underneath. Flip and cook for 2 to 3 minutes more. Repeat with the remaining batter, then serve.

Nutrition facts (per serving): 215 calories; 5 g fat; 330 mg sodium; 26 g carbs; 3 g fiber; 8 g sugar; 16 g protein

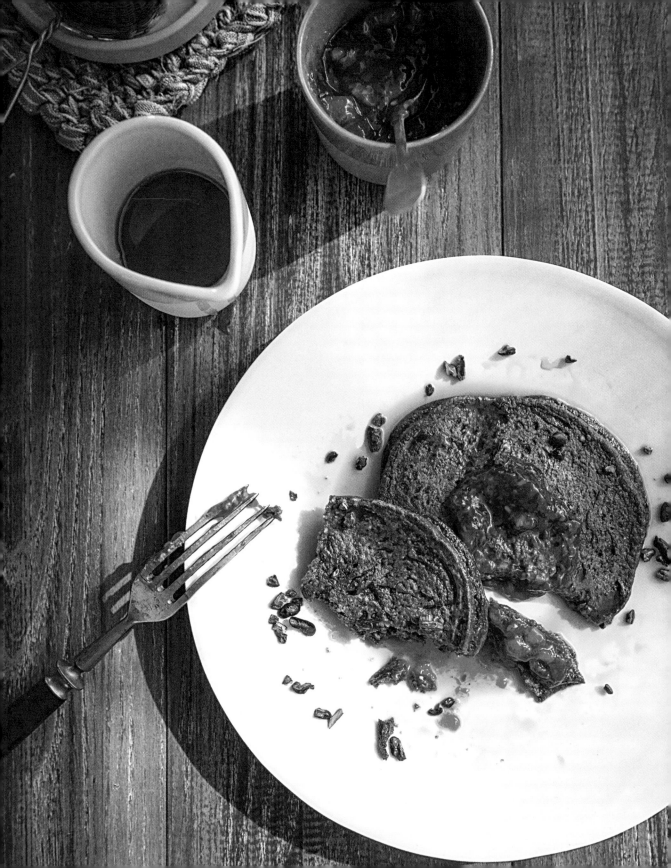

COCOA PROTEIN PANCAKES

GF

Makes 16 pancakes • Serving size: 6 pancakes

Eating chocolate pancakes when you're on a health kick is like the antithesis of what you'd imagine a diet to be. Unheard of! But it's true: You can have the decadence and fun of pancakes and still lose weight and eat virtuously! And because they're not drenched in syrup, you can eat them out of hand in the morning, almost like a soft cookie. I make four batches of these on a Sunday and freeze the extras in a baggie between pieces of waxed or parchment paper. To reheat, just toast them like a piece of bread and grab them on your way out.

2 tablespoons part-skim ricotta cheese

¼ cup liquid egg whites

¼ teaspoon sea salt

½ teaspoon pure vanilla extract

1 tablespoon unsweetened cocoa powder

¼ cup **Blueberry–Baby Spinach Base Blend** (page 98)

¼ cup low-fat milk (or unsweetened plant-based milk)

1 tablespoon pure maple syrup

⅔ cup rolled oats, finely ground (gluten free)

2 scoops unsweetened plain or vanilla protein powder

2 tablespoons cocoa nibs (optional)

Nonstick cooking spray

In a large bowl, whisk together all of the ingredients except the cocoa nibs. Mist a griddle or skillet with cooking spray and set over medium heat. Pour rounded tablespoons of batter into the pan and cook until bubbles begin to set around the edges and the pancakes are golden underneath. Sprinkle with cocoa nibs, if using, flip, and cook for 2 to 3 minutes more. Repeat with the remaining batter, then serve.

Nutrition facts (per serving): 210 calories; 6 g fat; 316 mg sodium; 27 g carbs; 5 g fiber; 7 g sugar; 14 g protein

BERRY DETOX SHAKE

• Makes 1 serving •

GF
V
* DF

You're already lovably familiar with this detox shake from the Reboot. I've included it again here because most people who have gone through the cleanse adopted this as their go-to breakfast—and kept sipping it long after the three days were up. It becomes habit because it satiates you for hours, and it has it all: good fat, good protein, and good fiber! This shake doesn't include a blend per se, because you're really just making one on the spot. It essentially contains my Blueberry–Baby Spinach Base Blend in unblended form.

1 cup frozen wild berries (blueberries, raspberries, or mixed berries)

½ cup plain low-fat Greek yogurt (or 1 scoop unsweetened plain or vanilla protein powder)

1 tablespoon ground flaxseed (or 1 teaspoon chia seeds)

1 cup loosely packed baby spinach

1 cup loosely packed baby kale

¼ ripe avocado

⅛ teaspoon ground cinnamon

1 to 2 teaspoons raw honey or pure maple syrup

1 cup cold filtered water

4 ice cubes

Place all of the ingredients into a high-powered blender and puree until smooth. Serve in a tall glass with a straw.

Nutrition facts: 279 calories; 9 g fat; 92 mg sodium; 38 g carbs; 13 g fiber; 17 g sugar; 15 g protein

* *(if using dairy-free protein powder)*

SUPER-GREENS DETOX SHAKE

GF
V
DF *

• *Makes 1 serving* •

This shake—which you also may remember from the Reboot—is my version of a green drink, only with loads of filling protein and fiber. Think of it as your insurance policy for the day: If things get crazy-busy and you don't eat your best, you'll know you've gotten your best meal of the day right here. Try this hack to make your A.M. prep take thirty seconds: Put all of the ingredients except the frozen fruit and ice in the blender and stash it in the fridge before you go to bed. In the morning, add the remaining ingredients and whiz it up. Note: This shake doesn't contain a blend because you're basically making one on the spot. Why would I make you blend something twice?

½ banana, ideally frozen

1 cup baby kale or baby
  spinach

1 tablespoon ground flaxseed

¼ ripe avocado

⅛ teaspoon ground cinnamon

½ cup plain low-fat Greek
  yogurt (or 1 scoop
  unsweetened plain or vanilla
  protein powder)

1 to 2 teaspoons raw honey or
  pure maple syrup

1 ½ cups filtered cold water

4 or 5 ice cubes

Place all of the ingredients into a high-powered blender and puree until smooth. Serve in a tall glass with a straw.

Nutrition facts: **268 calories; 9 g fat; 62 mg sodium; 37 g carbs; 8 g fiber; 20 g sugar; 15 g protein**

* *(if using dairy-free protein powder)*

DIY CREAM CHEESE

Makes 4 servings • Serving size: 2 tablespoons

I'm in love with this healthy cream cheese hack. I discovered it by accident one day when I was rushing and I dropped and cracked a container of Greek yogurt. I hastily stuck it in a bowl in the fridge. Later, I noticed that the liquid had strained out and the yogurt was even thicker than usual: It had taken on the consistency of cream cheese. Essentially, it's double-strained yogurt; Greek yogurt is already strained once, but this is even thicker. Now I use it in everything—as a cream cheese substitute, in dips in place of mayo and sour cream, even as a base for cupcake frosting!

Heaping ½ cup plain low-fat Greek yogurt

Place a strainer in a medium bowl and line it with 2 layers of paper towels. Add the yogurt and allow it to strain in the refrigerator for at least 30 minutes, or up to several days.

Nutrition facts (per serving): 18 calories; 0 g fat; 13 mg sodium; 1 g carbs; 0 g fiber; 1 g sugar; 3 g protein

— TRY IT ON —

Whole Wheat Bagel with Raspberry Cream Cheese (serves 4)

Stir 3 tablespoons Raspberry Base Blend into a batch of DIY cream cheese. Slice 2 whole wheat bagels in half, scoop out the centers, and toast. Top each bagel half with 2 tablespoons raspberry cream cheese and serve.

Nutrition facts (per serving): 288 calories; 1 g fat; 316 mg sodium; 55 g carbs; 6 g fiber; 4 g sugar; 17 g protein

WARM BUTTERNUT SQUASH–APPLE BREAKFAST SOUP

• Makes 1 serving •

Don't laugh at the idea of breakfast soup: The Scandinavians have been eating versions of this for ages. And it's the perfect thing on a chilly day when you don't want a cold smoothie. It's like autumn in a bowl.

1 cup **Butternut Squash–Apple Base Blend** (page 87)

Dash of ground cinnamon

Dash of sea salt

¼ cup low-fat milk or unsweetened plant-based milk

1 tablespoon pure maple syrup

2 tablespoons plain low-fat Greek yogurt

Warm the first 5 ingredients in a saucepan over medium heat. Pour into a bowl, stir in the yogurt, and serve.

Nutrition facts (per serving): 214 calories; 2 g fat; 56 mg sodium; 45 g carbs; 4 g fiber; 31 g sugar; 7 g protein

CHEESY KALE-BASIL SOUFFLÉ

• Makes 1 serving •

You can prep these soufflés in ramekins the night before, then either pop them into the toaster oven as you get ready in the morning or, if you're in a real rush, microwave them on high for 2 ½ minutes. Putting the Parm on top of the dish—instead of inside it—is a good trick. You taste it more and need to use less in the recipe.

Nonstick cooking spray

¼ cup **Sweet Pea–Baby Kale Base Blend** (page 91)

Handful of fresh basil leaves, finely chopped

2 large eggs

2 tablespoons low-fat milk

Pinch of sea salt

Freshly ground black pepper

2 tablespoons shredded Parmesan cheese

Preheat the oven to 400 degrees. Mist a ramekin (about 1 cup capacity) with cooking spray. In a small bowl, whisk together the blend, basil, eggs, and milk and season with salt and pepper. Pour the mixture into the ramekin and top with the cheese. Bake for about 18 minutes, until puffed and golden.

Nutrition facts (per serving): 217 calories; 12 g fat; 311 mg sodium; 10 g carbs; 2 g fiber; 2 g sugar; 18 g protein

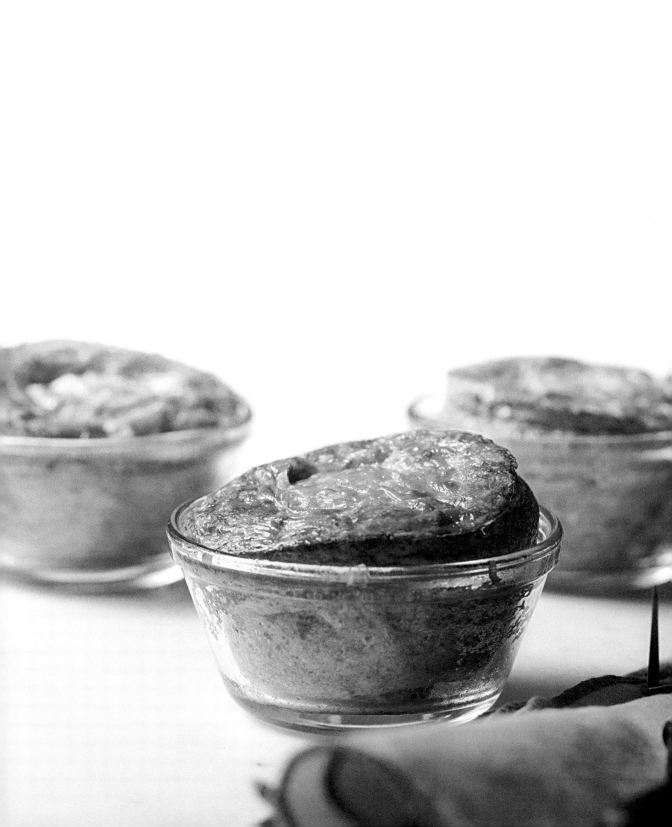

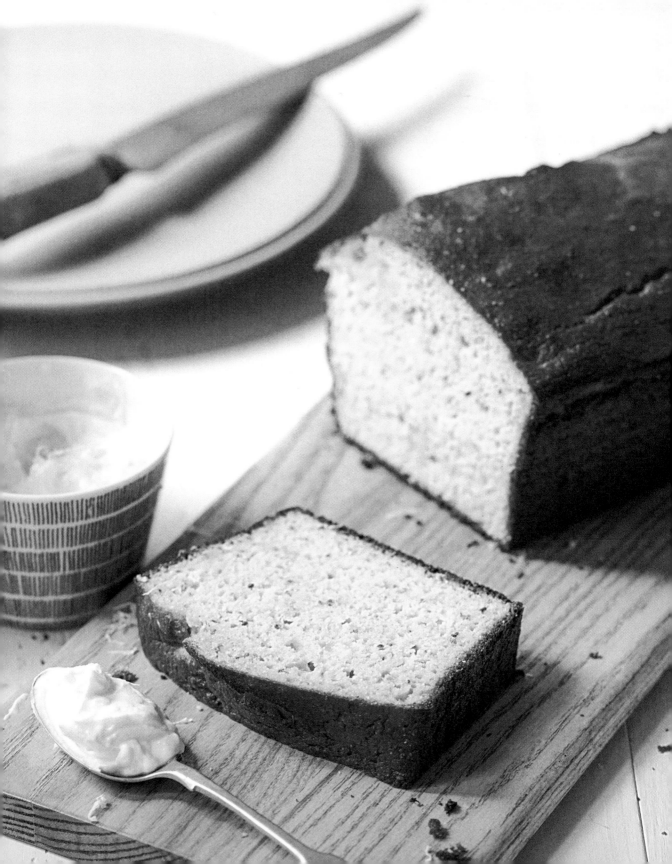

LEMON-CHIA QUICK BREAD

Makes 10 servings • Serving size: 1 1-inch-thick slice, plus 2 tablespoons DIY Cream Cheese

I always have this lemon quick bread on my counter. I make a batch on the weekend and have it all week with a lemony version of my original DIY Cream Cheese (page 128). It's light and nutritious and has whey protein for staying power. Note: Some lemon yogurts are super-high in added sugar, so read the labels.

For the quick bread
Zest and juice of 1 lemon

1 ½ tablespoons chia seeds

¼ cup canola oil

2 large eggs

¼ cup low-fat lemon Greek yogurt

¾ cup **Butternut Squash–Apple Base Blend** (page 87)

1 teaspoon pure vanilla extract

½ teaspoon sea salt

¼ cup raw honey

1 packet stevia (½ teaspoon)

1 tablespoon baking powder

½ cup plain, unsweetened whey protein (about 2 scoops)

1 cup unbleached white whole wheat flour

Nonstick cooking spray

For the lemon cream cheese
1 cup low-fat lemon Greek yogurt

Make the bread: Preheat the oven to 350 degrees. In a large bowl, whisk together the first 10 ingredients. Add the remaining dry ingredients and mix well. Mist a standard-size loaf pan with cooking spray. Pour the mixture into the pan and bake for about 40 minutes, until a toothpick placed in the center of the loaf comes out clean.

Meanwhile, make the lemon cream cheese: Place a strainer in a medium bowl and line it with 2 layers of paper towels. Add the yogurt and allow it to strain in the refrigerator for at least 30 minutes, or up to several days. Top each slice of bread with 2 tablespoons of the lemon cream cheese.

Nutrition facts (per serving): **201 calories; 8 g fat; 304 mg sodium; 22 g carbs; 3 g fiber; 11 g sugar; 11 g protein**

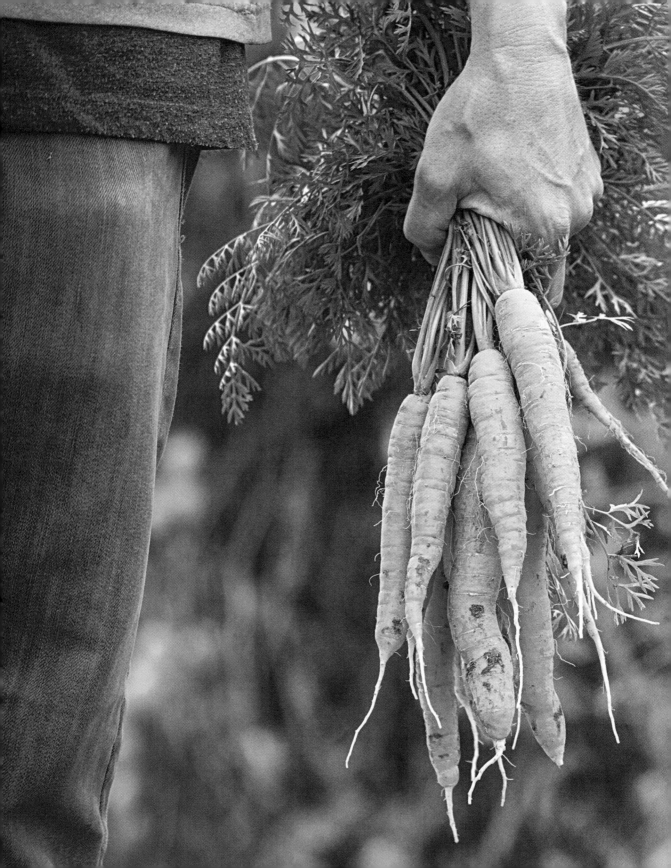

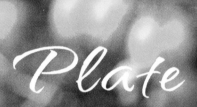

Plate

Main Courses and Lighter Lunches

Pizza? Check! Pasta Bolognese? Check! Creamy, satisfying soups? Check! You'll find all sorts of delicious, good-for-you lunch and dinner recipes here—which have, of course, been lightened up with my blends. The handy chart below lists each meal with the blend it uses, as well as other blends you can sub in. It helps you figure out which recipe to make based on whatever blends you have on hand. Enjoy!

THE DISH	THE BASE BLEND
Warm Green Basil Blend	Broccoli-Pea-Spinach Base Blend (or any Green Base Blend)
Thai-Style Blend	Sweet Pea Base Blend (or any Green Base Blend)
Tex-Mex Blend	Black Bean–Blueberry–Baby Kale Base Blend
Spring Sweet Pea Soup	Sweet Pea Base Blend
Quinoa-Crusted Chicken Parm with Roasted Green Beans	Carrot–Sweet Potato Base Blend
Southwestern Turkey Burger with Crunchy Jicama "Fries"	Black Bean–Blueberry–Baby Kale Base Blend (or Blueberry–Baby Spinach Base Blend)
Crunchy Kale-Crust Pizza	White Bean Base Blend (or any White Base Blend)
Parisian Tuna Salad	White Bean Base Blend (or Chickpea-Zucchini Base Blend)
Seared Salmon with Dill Sauce	Broccoli-Pea-Spinach Base Blend (or any Green Base Blend)
Creamy Tomato-Basil Soup	Cauliflower Base Blend (or any White Base Blend)
Baja Veggie Tacos	Black Bean–Blueberry–Baby Kale Base Blend
Chicken Satay with Coconut-Lime Peanut Dipping Sauce	Carrot–Sweet Potato Base Blend
Raspberry-Glazed Pork Tenderloin with Roasted Broccoli	Raspberry-Beet Base Blend (or Raspberry Base Blend)
Zucchini Pasta Piccata	Chickpea-Zucchini Base Blend (or any White Base Blend)
Single-Serve Mac and Cheese	Carrot–Sweet Potato Base Blend
Southwestern Burrito Bowl	Black Bean–Blueberry–Baby Kale Base Blend

THE DISH	THE BASE BLEND
Miso-Ginger Cod in Parchment	Carrot–Sweet Potato Base Blend
Citrus-Herb Roasted Turkey with Mushroom Gravy	White Bean Base Blend (or Chickpea-Zucchini Base Blend)
Pesto Pasta with Roasted Shrimp	Broccoli-Pea-Spinach Base Blend (or any Green Base Blend)
Not Your Mom's (Turkey) Meat Loaf	Black Bean–Blueberry–Baby Kale Base Blend (or Blueberry–Baby Spinach Base Blend)
Meaty Mushroom Bolognese	Carrot–Sweet Potato Base Blend
Crunchy Tofu Sticks with Small-Batch Ketchup	Carrot–Sweet Potato Base Blend
Miso-Kale Noodle Bowl	Chickpea-Zucchini Base Blend (or any White Base Blend)
Coconut Corn Chowder with Cilantro and Lime	Cauliflower Base Blend (or any White Base Blend)
Curried Chicken Salad-Stuffed Pitas	White Bean Base Blend (or Chickpea-Zucchini Base Blend)
(Not) Forbidden Rice Salad with Raspberry-Beet Vinaigrette	Raspberry-Beet Base Blend (or any Red Base Blend)
DIY Salads: Miso-Ginger Dressing	Carrot–Sweet Potato Base Blend
DIY Salads: All Hail Eggless Caesar Dressing	Cauliflower Base Blend (or any White Base Blend)
DIY Salads: Even Greener Goddess Dressing	Sweet Pea Base Blend (or any Green Base Blend)
DIY Salads: Creamy Feta Dressing	Cauliflower Base Blend
DIY Salads: Revamped Russian Dressing	White Bean Base Blend (or Chickpea-Zucchini Base Blend)
DIY Salads: Raspberry-Beet Vinaigrette	Raspberry-Beet Base Blend (or Beet Base Blend)
DIY Pasta Dinners: Creamy No-Tomato Pasta Sauce	Carrot–Sweet Potato Base Blend
DIY Pasta Dinners: Pistachio Power Pesto	Broccoli-Pea-Spinach Base Blend (or any Green Base Blend)
DIY Pasta Dinners: Make-It-in-Minutes Marinara Sauce	Carrot–Sweet Potato Base Blend

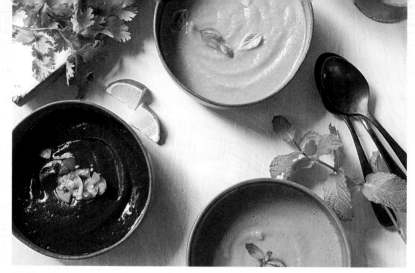

1-MINUTE MEALS

These super speedy recipes are essentially doctored-up versions of my Base Blends. You add a couple of ingredients and the blend transforms into a satisfying meal—like the ones you made during the Reboot. I got this idea from my blends community. Many of them were enjoying the blends more straight up—with just a few herbs or spices thrown in to make it a delicious meal all on its own. Love it! It's fast, it's convenient (you can use a blend you already have ready to go) and there's something simple and wholesome about it.

GF
V

WARM GREEN BASIL BLEND

• *Makes 1 serving* •

1 cup **Broccoli-Pea-Spinach Base Blend**
(page 90)

1 tablespoon extra-virgin olive oil

A few finely minced fresh basil leaves

Pinch of sea salt

1 tablespoon freshly grated Parmesan
cheese

Warm all of the ingredients in a small saucepan over medium-low heat, mixing well to combine, and serve.

Nutrition facts: **223 calories; 16 g fat; 195 mg sodium; 15 g carbs; 4 g fiber; 4 g sugar; 9 g protein**

THAI-STYLE BLEND

• *Makes 1 serving* •

1 cup **Sweet Pea Base Blend** (page 92)

1 tablespoon extra-virgin olive oil

2 tablespoons light coconut milk

Pinch of sea salt

Handful of finely minced fresh mint leaves

Warm all of the ingredients in a small saucepan over medium-low heat, mixing well to combine, and serve.

Nutrition facts: 248 calories; 15 g fat; 305 mg sodium; 19 g carbs; 6 g fiber; 7 g sugar; 8 g protein

TEX-MEX BLEND

• *Makes 1 serving* •

1 cup **Black Bean–Blueberry–Baby Kale Base Blend** (page 100)

⅛ teaspoon ground cumin

¼ teaspoon chili powder

2 to 3 tablespoons salsa, ideally fresh

Pinch of sea salt

Warm all of the ingredients in a small saucepan over medium-low heat, mixing well to combine, and serve.

Nutrition facts: 256 calories; 1 g fat; 260 mg sodium; 49 g carbs; 15 g fiber; 8 g sugar; 14 g protein

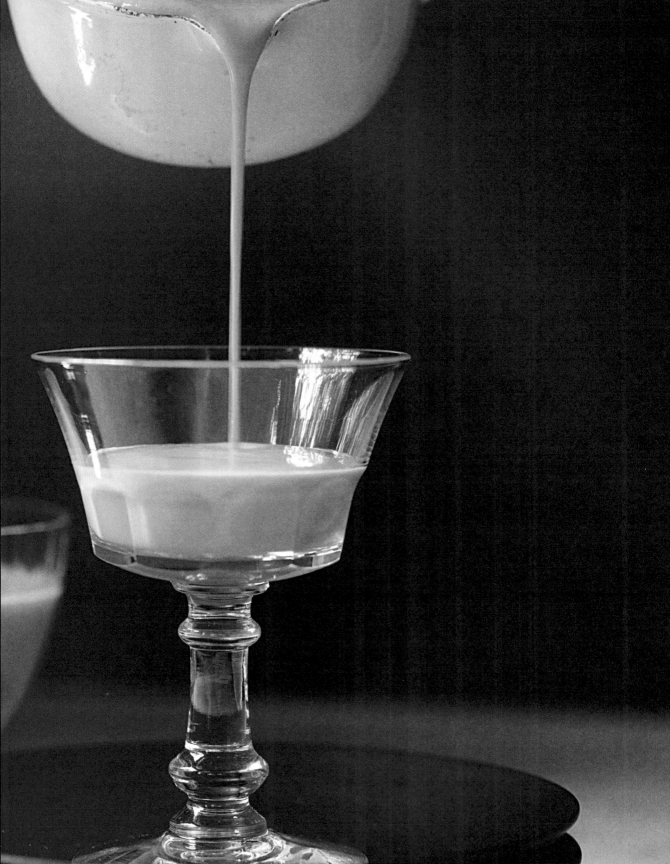

SPRING SWEET PEA SOUP

Makes 4 servings • Serving size: about 1 ¹/₂ cups

This soup is so fresh and incredibly easy to make. It's also good hot or cold, so you can enjoy it year-round. If you don't have Sweet Pea Base Blend on hand, you can just pour boiling water over 6 cups of frozen peas and then whiz everything up in the blender.

3 ½ cups **Sweet Pea Base Blend** (page 92)

1 ½ cups low-sodium vegetable broth (or chicken broth)

½ cup low-fat milk or unsweetened plant-based milk

a few fresh mint or basil leaves

¼ teaspoon sea salt

1 tablespoon avocado oil or extra-virgin olive oil

Puree all of the ingredients until smooth. Serve warm or chilled.

Nutrition facts (per serving): 199 calories; 4 g fat; 468 mg sodium; 28 g carbs; 9 g fiber; 9 g sugar; 13 g protein

* *(if using vegetable broth)*

QUINOA-CRUSTED CHICKEN PARM WITH ROASTED GREEN BEANS

Makes 4 servings • Serving size: 3 ounces chicken, plus sauce and 1 cup beans

This is a super-simple way of breading chicken that is less messy and time-consuming than the traditional method. The quinoa adds great crunch and is way better for you—Fiber! Iron!—than refined flour and white bread crumbs.

For the chicken

½ cup uncooked quinoa

¼ teaspoon dried oregano

A few turns of freshly ground black pepper

4 4-ounce boneless, skinless chicken breasts, pounded thin

1 ½ cups Make-It-in-Minutes Marinara Sauce (page 191), or 1 cup of your favorite store-bought sauce with ⅓ cup **Carrot–Sweet Potato Base Blend** (page 86)

⅓ cup shredded part-skim mozzarella cheese

3 tablespoons freshly grated Parmesan cheese

For the green beans

4 cups string beans, ends trimmed

½ tablespoon extra-virgin olive oil

Pinch of red pepper flakes

Sea salt and freshly ground black pepper

Make the chicken: Preheat the oven to 400 degrees. Pulse the dry quinoa in a food processor for about 30 seconds, until it resembles flour. Rinse it in a fine-mesh strainer to remove the bitter coating; drain well and place the damp quinoa into a gallon-size resealable plastic bag. Add the oregano and pepper to the bag and shake to mix. Add the chicken pieces and shake again to coat evenly.

Spread ¾ cup of the sauce on the bottom of a 13 x 9-inch glass or ceramic baking dish. Lay the breaded cutlets on top of the sauce, side by side. Pour the remaining sauce over the chicken and top each cutlet evenly with the mozzarella and Parmesan. Bake, uncovered, for 25 to 30 minutes, or until the chicken is cooked through and the cheese is lightly browned and bubbly.

Meanwhile, make the beans: Put the beans, oil, and red pepper flakes on a baking sheet and toss to combine. Season with salt and pepper. Roast them alongside the chicken during the last 10 minutes of cooking, until they're lightly browned and crisp.

Nutrition facts (per serving): 440 calories; 13 g fat; 338 mg sodium; 36 g carbs; 7 g fiber; 4 g sugar; 45 g protein

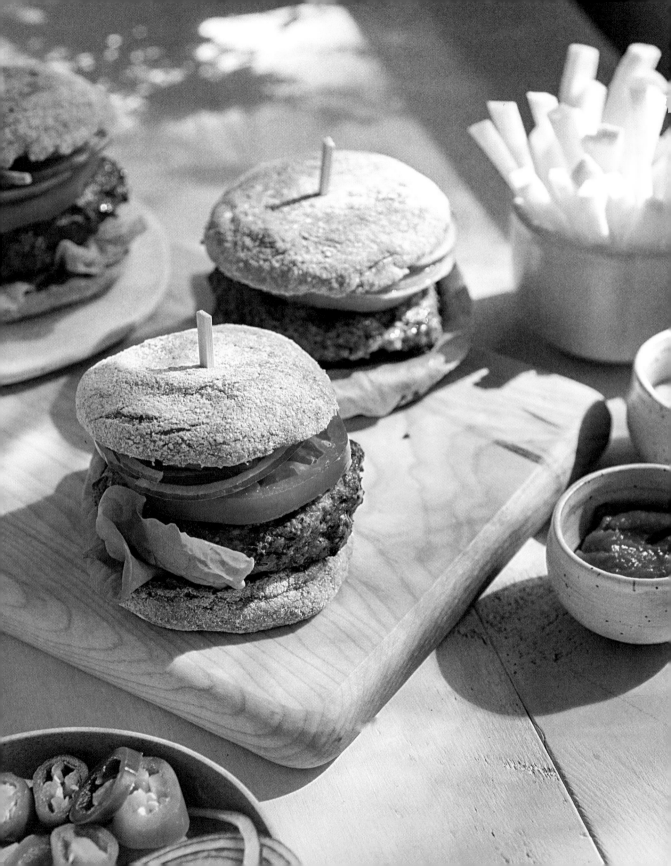

SOUTHWESTERN TURKEY BURGERS WITH CRUNCHY JICAMA "FRIES"

Makes 4 servings • Serving size: 1 burger, plus ¹/₂ cup jicama sticks

I'm usually not a fan of turkey burgers; they're so bland and hockey-puck-like. The spices in my version punch up the flavor and the Black Bean–Blueberry–Baby Kale Base Blend adds moistness and a "beefiness" to the burgers. Note: Ground dark meat turkey can have even more fat than ground beef, so read the labels and make sure you grab the lean kind.

6 tablespoons **Black Bean–Blueberry–Baby Kale Base Blend** (page 100)

1 teaspoon Worcestershire sauce

½ teaspoon chili powder

½ teaspoon onion powder

⅛ teaspoon sea salt

A few turns of freshly ground black pepper

½ cup ground oats (blitzed in a food processor) or ground flaxseed

12 ounces lean ground turkey

4 whole grain English muffins

Lettuce, onion, tomatoes, pickled jalapeños (optional toppings)

2 cups jicama sticks, cut into ½-inch-thick fry-like pieces

In a large bowl, whisk together the blend, Worcestershire sauce, chili powder, and onion powder and season with salt and pepper. Add the oats and turkey and mix to combine. Form 4 equal-size balls and gently press them into ½-inch-thick patties. Grill for 7 to 8 minutes per side, until cooked through. Serve on toasted English muffins with the toppings as desired, and serve the raw jicama sticks on the side.

Nutrition facts (per serving): 317 calories; 4 g fat; 358 mg sodium; 43 g carbs; 8 g fiber; 6 g sugar; 29 g protein

CRUNCHY KALE-CRUST PIZZA

Makes 4 servings • Serving size: 1 pizza

I'm always on the lookout for a pizza crust that isn't just a refined carb fest—and this is one of the best I've ever had. It's incredibly good for you in and of itself, not just a delivery system for the sauce and cheese. What's not to love?

1 tablespoon tomato paste

⅓ cup chopped fresh basil leaves

½ cup egg whites (about 3 eggs)

¼ teaspoon dried oregano

1 cup finely chopped baby kale

¼ cup **White Bean Base Blend** (page 83)

3 tablespoons grated Parmesan cheese

¼ cup gluten-free flour

Nonstick cooking spray

¾ cup Make-It-in-Minutes Marinara Sauce (page 191), or your favorite pizza or pasta sauce*

1 cup grated part-skim mozzarella

In a medium bowl, whisk together the first 7 ingredients. Add the flour and mix well to combine. Mist an 8-inch skillet with the cooking spray and place over medium-high heat. Add ¼ cup batter and shake the pan to make the crust spread out. Cook for a few minutes, until the bottom is crisp and browned, then flip and cook for another few minutes. Repeat with the remaining batter, re-spraying the pan between batches (the batter makes 4 crusts).

Preheat the broiler. Place the crusts on a baking sheet and divide the sauce and mozzarella equally among them. Broil for a few minutes until the cheese is browned and bubbly.

* Check out my Sneaky Chef pasta sauces with hidden veggies (thesneakychef.com).

Nutrition facts (per serving): 161 calories; 8 g fat; 277 mg sodium; 13 g carbs; 2 g fiber; 1 g sugar; 14 g protein

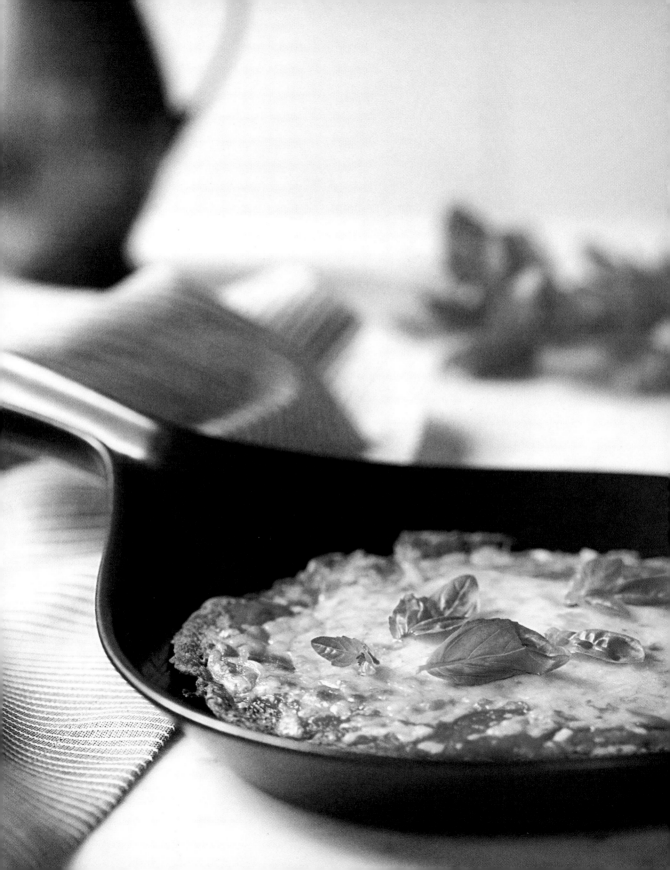

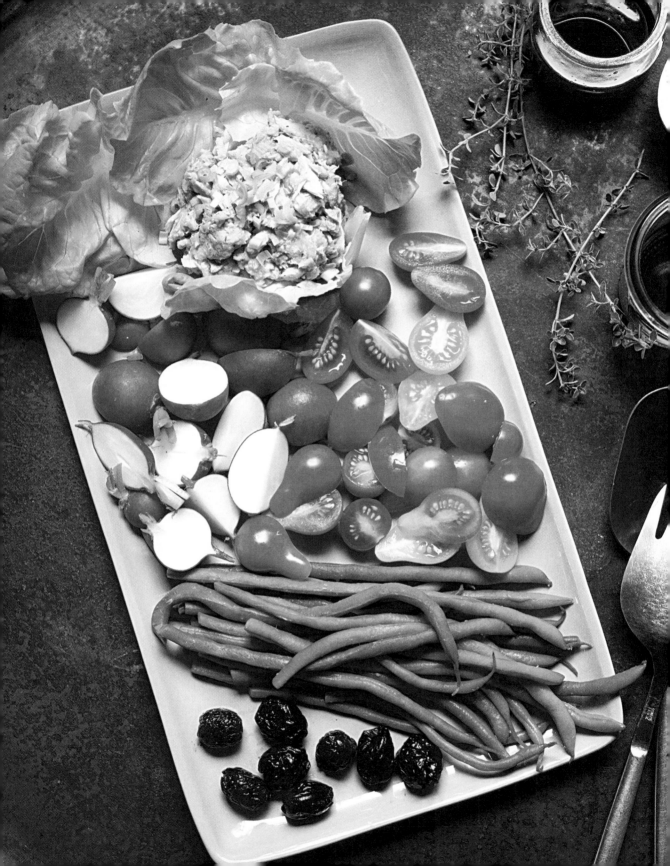

PARISIAN TUNA SALAD

GF

Makes 2 servings • Serving size: about ³/₄ cup

Here, White Bean Base Blend stands in for mayo, providing the creaminess you want, but in a fiber- and phytonutrient-rich way. And get this: One serving of this blend has just 39 calories and 0 grams of fat; the same amount of mayo has 180 calories and 20 fat grams. It's more proof that one small swap can make an enormous difference in your diet. Make this mayo swap just twice a week and you'll effortlessly drop 5 pounds this year!

¼ cup **White Bean Base Blend** (page 83)

1 tablespoon chopped fresh thyme, or ½ teaspoon dried thyme

1 4- to 5-ounce can chunk light tuna in water

1 cup raw haricots verts, trimmed and blanched

8 niçoise olives, pitted and chopped

½ cup radishes, halved

½ cup grape tomatoes, halved

½ tablespoon extra-virgin olive oil

1 tablespoon balsamic vinegar

Sea salt and freshly ground black pepper

In a large bowl, add the blend, thyme, and tuna and fold to combine. Place the tuna mixture on a large plate with the haricots verts, olives, radishes, and tomatoes. In a small bowl, whisk together the olive oil and balsamic vinegar, and drizzle over the veggies. Season with salt and pepper to taste and serve.

Nutrition facts (per serving): 206 calories; 8 g fat; 250 mg sodium; 17 g carbs; 4 g fiber; 2 g sugar; 17 g protein

SEARED SALMON WITH DILL SAUCE

Makes 4 servings • Serving size: About 5 ounces salmon, plus 1 cup baby kale

I prefer wild salmon to farm raised because it has fewer toxins, such as PCBs. It's more expensive, but here's a tip: Frozen salmon is cheaper than fresh. It thaws quickly in the fridge and sometimes I even throw it into the pan or oven while it's still frozen. Just be careful not to overcook fish or it will dry out.

¼ cup **Broccoli-Pea-Spinach Base Blend** (page 90)

3 tablespoons minced fresh dill

2 teaspoons freshly squeezed lemon juice

2 tablespoons plain low-fat Greek yogurt

4 wild salmon fillets (1 ¼ to 1 ½ pounds total)

1 tablespoon extra-virgin olive oil

4 cups baby kale, rinsed and spun dry

Lemon wedges, for serving

Whisk the blend, dill, lemon juice, and yogurt together in a medium bowl. Place a sauté pan over medium-high heat. Brush the salmon with the oil and place skin side up in the pan. Sear for 5 minutes, then flip and cook for about 5 minutes more, until just cooked through. Divide the baby kale among 4 plates and place the hot salmon over to wilt it. Top each piece of fish with 2 tablespoons of the dill sauce and serve with lemon wedges.

Nutrition facts (per serving): 305 calories; 16 g fat; 96 mg sodium; 6 g carbs; 1 g fiber; 1 g sugar; 33 g protein

CREAMY TOMATO-BASIL SOUP

GF V DF *

Makes 3 servings • Serving size: 2 cups

Cauliflower Base Blend stands in for heavy cream in this homey soup—a trick you can use to add body to any creamy soup. I like to use whole canned or boxed tomatoes, rather than the crushed or pureed kind, because food manufacturers tend to use higher-quality produce for them—who knew? If you want to make this meal more substantial, add a slice of whole grain bread.

2 tablespoons extra-virgin olive oil

1 medium Vidalia onion, diced

1 garlic clove, minced

1 28-ounce box whole tomatoes, with juice

½ cup low-sodium vegetable broth (or chicken broth)

½ cup **Cauliflower Base Blend** (page 84)

¼ cup chopped fresh basil

Sea salt and freshly ground black pepper

Heat the oil in a medium pot over medium heat. Add the onion and cook for 5 to 6 minutes, until translucent. Add the garlic and cook for 1 minute. Add the tomatoes and their juice, the broth, and the blend and simmer, uncovered, for 15 minutes. Stir in the basil and season with salt and pepper to taste. Carefully pour the soup into a high-powered blender and puree until smooth. Serve.

Nutrition facts (per serving): 177 calories; 9 g fat; 158 mg sodium; 23 g carbs; 7 g fiber; 13 g sugar; 4 g protein

* *(if made with vegetable broth)*

BAJA VEGGIE TACOS

Makes 4 servings • Serving size: 2 tacos

Romaine lettuce is a clever swap for taco shells: The leaves are the perfect shape and still give you great crunch. (Choose sturdy, curved inner leaves that will hold up to the filling and toppings.) The spice-spiked Black Bean–Blueberry–Baby Kale Base Blend is like a refried bean substitute, only so much healthier: Each serving delivers more than one third of your daily fiber requirement.

8 large leaves of romaine, rinsed and patted dry

1 cup **Black Bean–Blueberry–Baby Kale Base Blend** (page 100)

2 tablespoons salsa or tomato paste

1 teaspoon chili powder

¼ teaspoon onion powder

¼ teaspoon dried oregano

¼ teaspoon ground cumin

¼ teaspoon garlic powder

¼ teaspoon sea salt

Pinch of cayenne pepper, or more to taste

¼ cup chopped tomatoes

¼ cup frozen corn, thawed

¼ cup shredded sharp cheddar cheese

¼ cup chopped fresh cilantro

Lay 2 lettuce leaves on each plate. In a medium bowl, whisk together the blend, salsa, and all of the spices. Spread 2 tablespoons of the bean mixture on each lettuce leaf. Top each taco with 1 tablespoon each of tomatoes, corn, cheese, and cilantro and serve.

Nutrition facts (per serving): 231 calories; 4 g fat; 164 mg sodium; 39 g carbs; 13 g fiber; 8 g sugar; 14 g protein

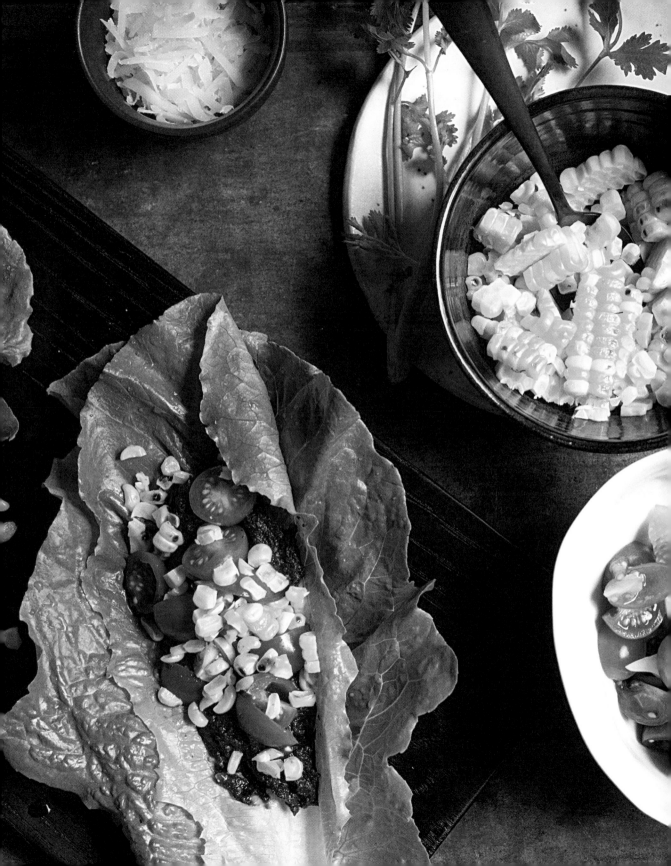

CHICKEN SATAY WITH COCONUT-LIME PEANUT DIPPING SAUCE

Makes 4 servings • Serving size: 3 skewers, plus veggies and garnish

Anything on a skewer turns an everyday meal into a party. The coconut and lime in this recipe add a Thai twist to traditional peanut sauce. Ordinarily, this dipping sauce is super-heavy, but the Carrot–Sweet Potato Base Blend and coconut milk lighten it up. Note: If you're allergic to peanuts, you can sub in a peanut butter alternative like my Sneaky Chef No-Nut Butter (thesneakychef.com).

For the peanut dipping sauce

¼ cup smooth, natural peanut butter

½ cup light coconut milk

6 tablespoons **Carrot–Sweet Potato Base Blend** (page 86)

4 teaspoons reduced-sodium soy sauce (or gluten-free tamari)

2 tablespoons freshly squeezed lime juice

⅛ to ¼ teaspoon red pepper flakes

2 teaspoons minced garlic

For the chicken

Juice of 1 orange

Juice of 1 lime

12 ounces boneless, skinless chicken breasts, cut into 12 strips

Peanut dipping sauce (below)

12 wooden skewers

2 cups shredded cabbage

2 tablespoons chopped green onions, for garnish

2 tablespoons chopped peanuts, for garnish

Make the sauce: Whisk together all of the sauce ingredients in a large bowl.

Make the chicken: Pour the orange and lime juice and half of the peanut sauce into a large resealable plastic bag. Add the chicken strips, squeeze out the air, seal the bag tightly, and shake to distribute the marinade. Allow the chicken to

* *(if using tamari)*

marinate in the refrigerator for at least 1 hour and up to 24 hours, turning the bag occasionally.

Soak the skewers in water for 30 minutes, to prevent burning. Preheat a grill (or grill pan) to medium-high. Remove the chicken (discard the marinade) and push 1 skewer through the long end of each chicken strip. Grill the chicken for 3 to 5 minutes per side, until cooked through. Place ½ cup of the cabbage on each plate and top with warm chicken skewers; sprinkle with green onions and peanuts. Serve each with 2 tablespoons of the remaining peanut dipping sauce on the side, for dunking.

Nutrition facts (per serving): 301 calories; 14 g fat; 267 mg sodium; 12 g carbs; 3 g fiber; 5 g sugar; 32 g protein

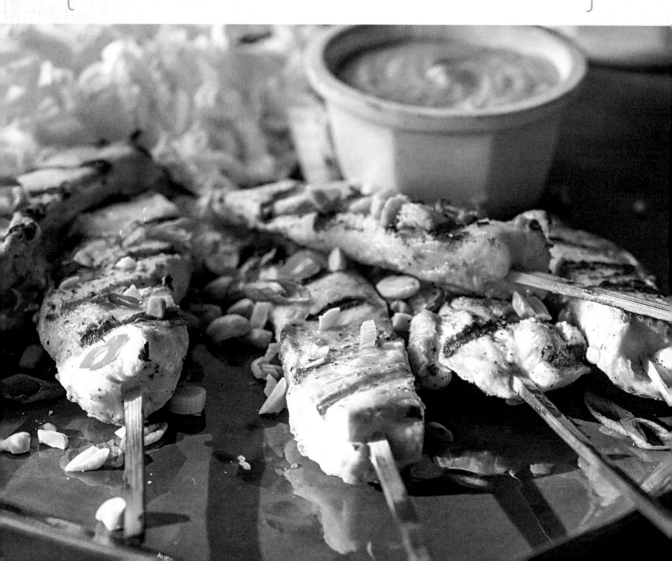

RASPBERRY-GLAZED PORK TENDERLOIN WITH ROASTED BROCCOLI

Makes 4 servings • Serving size: 4 ounces pork, plus sauce and veggies

Pork tenderloin is as lean as boneless, skinless chicken breast; and the sweet-savory sauce just makes this whole dish crazy good.

For the pork

½ cup **Raspberry-Beet Base Blend** (page 94)

¼ cup balsamic vinegar

1 tablespoon raw honey

¼ teaspoon sea salt

1 pork tenderloin (about 1 pound)

For the broccoli

8 cups broccoli florets

1 tablespoon extra-virgin olive oil

Sea salt and freshly ground black pepper

2 large shallots, peeled and thinly sliced

Make the pork: In a medium bowl, whisk together the blend, vinegar, honey, and salt. Pour half of the sauce into a large resealable plastic bag; refrigerate remaining sauce until ready to use. Place the pork in the bag, squeeze out the air, seal it tightly, and shake to distribute the sauce. Allow the pork to marinate in the refrigerator for at least 30 minutes and up to 24 hours, turning the bag occasionally. Remove the pork and place in a foil-lined baking dish; pour the sauce it was marinating in over top.

Make the broccoli: Place the broccoli on a baking sheet and toss with the oil. Season with salt and pepper and sprinkle the shallots over top.

Preheat the broiler.

Place the pork on the baking sheet alongside the broccoli. Broil the pork and broccoli 5 to 6 inches from the heat source for 15 to 20 minutes, turning once halfway through cooking, until the meat registers 145 degrees at the thickest part and the broccoli is crisp and browned around the edges. Allow the pork to rest for 5 minutes, then slice and divide it among plates. Serve each with 2 tablespoons of the reserved sauce and a quarter of the broccoli.

Nutrition facts (per serving): 357 calories; 9 g fat; 256 mg sodium; 31 g carbs; 13 g fiber; 14 g sugar; 44 g protein

ZUCCHINI PASTA PICCATA

Makes 4 servings • Serving size: About 3 cups

Here, simple "spiralized" zucchini subs for whole grain pasta. It's fun twirling the "noodles" on your fork, and zucchini is practically a free food. It's one of the lightest, lowest-calorie veggies out there—so you can have a huge, satisfying mound of it. You can pick up one of those super-trendy spiralizers for around $10, or make the zucchini noodles yourself with a vegetable peeler (see the how-to below).

2 tablespoons extra-virgin olive oil, divided

1 cup low-sodium chicken broth, divided (or Bone Broth, page 56)

12 ounces boneless, skinless chicken breasts, cut into cubes

¼ cup freshly squeezed lemon juice

3 teaspoons capers, drained

½ cup **Chickpea-Zucchini Base Blend** (page 82)

2 medium zucchini

Sea salt and freshly ground black pepper

½ cup chopped fresh flat-leaf parsley

Place a large skillet over medium-high heat. Add 1 tablespoon of the oil and 3 tablespoons of the broth. Add about half of the chicken (don't crowd the pan) and cook for 5 minutes per side, until lightly browned; transfer to a plate. Heat the remaining tablespoon of oil and 3 tablespoons of the broth and cook the remaining chicken. Transfer the chicken to the plate. Add the remaining ½ cup broth to the pan, along with the lemon juice, capers, and the blend, and bring to a broil, scraping the brown bits from the bottom of the pan. Return the chicken to the pan and simmer for 5 minutes.

Meanwhile, bring a kettle of water to a boil. Make noodles (or "zoodles") out of the zucchini using a spiralizer or vegetable peeler. (If using a peeler, run it lengthwise down the zucchini until you get down to the seeds; discard that center part). Place the zucchini strands in a large fine-mesh strainer. Pour the boiling water over the zoodles to quick-cook them to al dente. Place about 2 cups of the zoodles on each plate, along with one quarter of the chicken mixture. Season with salt and pepper to taste, sprinkle with parsley, and serve.

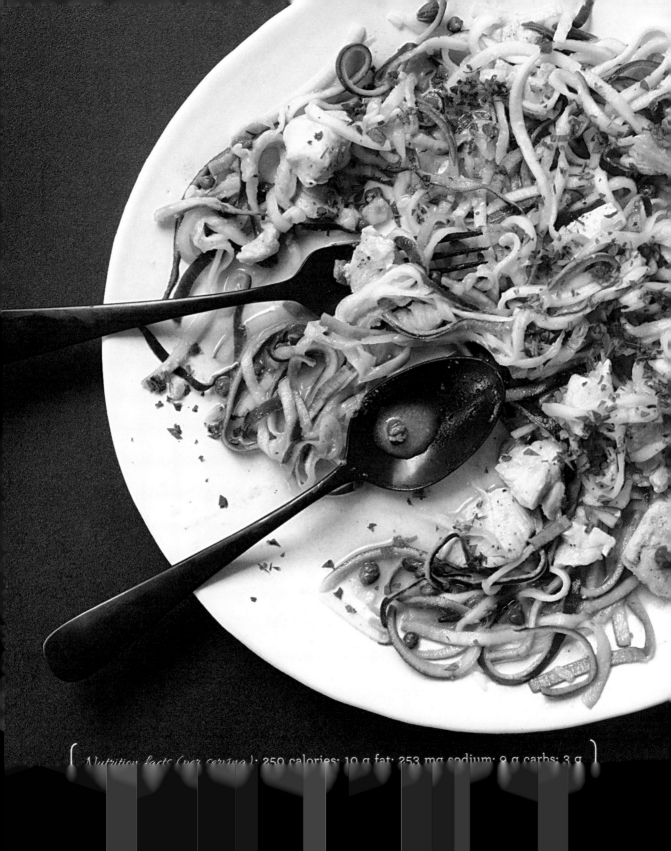

Nutrition facts (per serving): 250 calories; 10 g fat; 253 mg sodium; 9 g carbs; 3 g

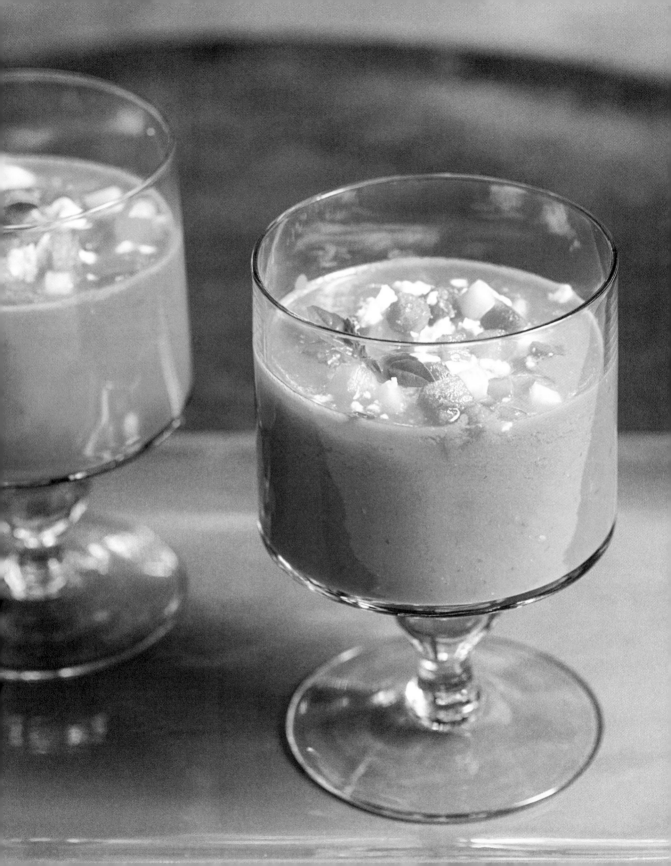

CHILLED WATERMELON-CUCUMBER GAZPACHO

Makes 4 servings • Serving size: About 1 cup

This soup is my go-to during the summer. It's so satisfying and fresh and cool—and, let me tell you, it's way easier than chopping a salad for yourself. (The gazpacho doesn't use a blend because I consider the whole thing to be one big blend.) I like a chunkier texture, but if you like it totally smooth just blitz all of the ingredients for the soup together. For a heartier meal, add ¼ avocado, diced; it adds just 69 calories and is a delicious add-on.

2 cups seeded and roughly chopped watermelon, plus 1 cup diced watermelon for garnish

1 ½ tablespoons extra-virgin olive oil

1 ½ tablespoons red or white wine vinegar

1 seedless cucumber, peeled and roughly chopped

12 grape tomatoes (or 1 large ripe beefsteak tomato, in season)

1 yellow or red bell pepper, seeded and roughly chopped

Handful of fresh basil leaves

Sea salt and freshly ground black pepper

¼ cup crumbled feta cheese, for garnish

Puree the 2 cups watermelon with the oil, vinegar, and half of the cucumber until almost smooth. Add the remaining cucumber, the tomatoes, bell pepper, and basil and pulse until combined, but still slightly chunky. Season with salt and pepper to taste and serve, topping each bowl with 2 tablespoons of the diced watermelon and 1 tablespoon of the feta.

Nutrition facts (per serving): **154 calories; 9 g fat; 152 mg sodium; 16 g carbs; 2 g fiber; 9 g sugar; 5 g protein**

SINGLE-SERVE
MAC AND CHEESE

• *Makes 1 serving* •

The secret to this totally diet-friendly version of mac and cheese? The blend and cauliflower florets add volume—so you get to eat more—and I use super-flavorful cheeses. Result: A decadent meal that has three times fewer calories than standard mac and cheese.

¾ cup cooked whole grain
   rotini pasta

⅓ cup **Carrot–Sweet Potato
   Base Blend** (page 86)

1 egg white

⅛ teaspoon mustard powder

½ ounce goat cheese,
   crumbled

1 tablespoon low-fat milk

1 heaping tablespoon sharp
   cheddar cheese

½ cup chopped cauliflower
   florets

Pinch of sea salt and freshly
   ground black pepper

1 tablespoon freshly grated
   Parmesan cheese

Preheat the oven to 400 degrees. In a large bowl, mix all of the ingredients except the Parmesan together. Pour into an ovenproof bowl, sprinkle the Parmesan over the top, and bake for 20 minutes, until the top is browned and bubbly.

Nutrition facts (per serving): 302 calories; 7 g fat; 287 mg sodium; 41 g carbs; 6 g fiber; 6 g sugar; 20 g protein

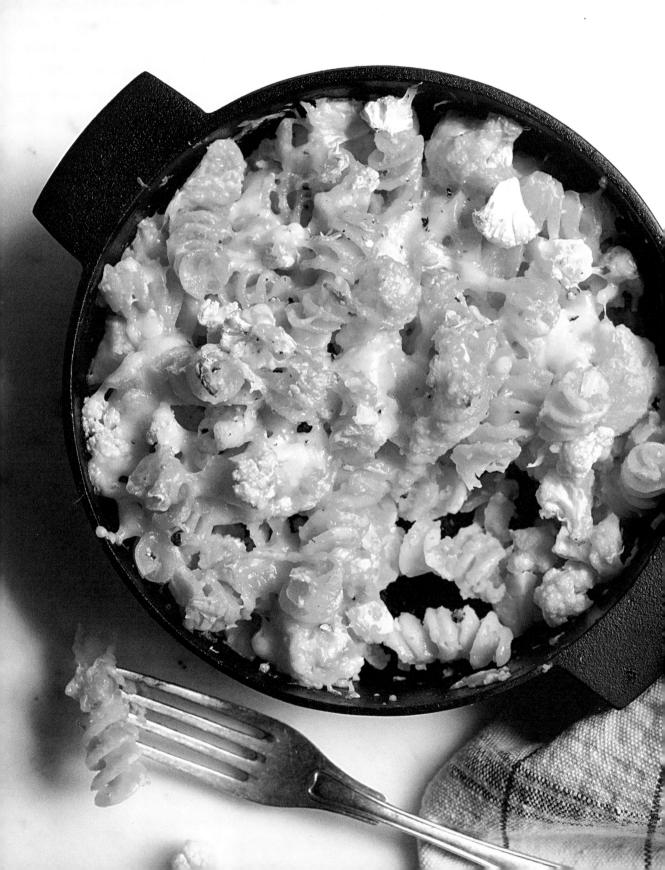

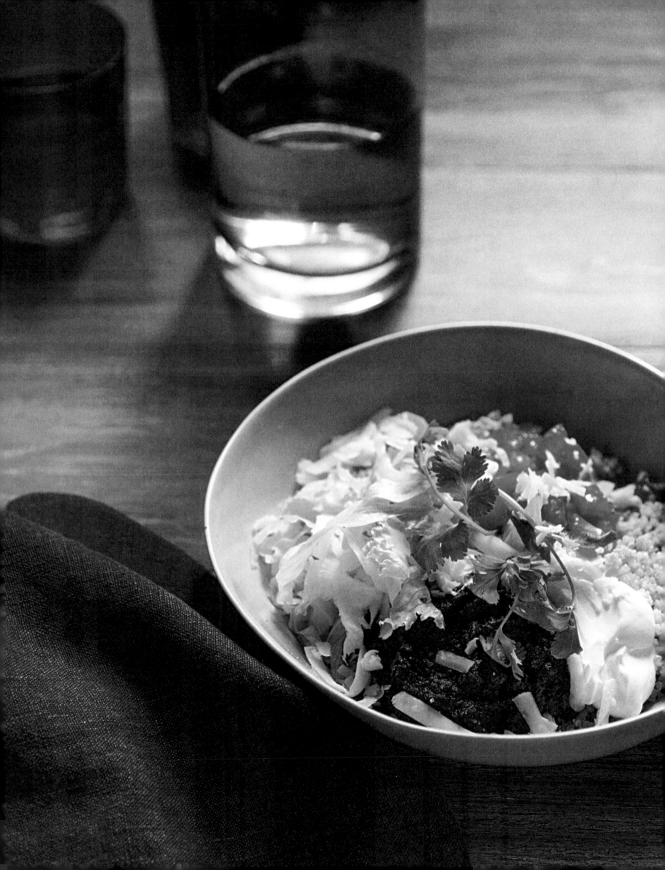

SOUTHWESTERN BURRITO BOWL ⑥Ⓕ

Makes 4 servings • Serving size: About 1 cup

Burrito bowls are deceptive. You think that by skipping the wrap, the meal is healthier and lower in calories. But really, you're getting several servings of white rice, loads of cheese, and lard-laden refried beans. Not this one, which stars my Black Bean–Blueberry–Baby Kale Base Blend as a delicious substitute for refried beans.

1 cup **Black Bean–Blueberry–Baby Kale Base Blend** (page 100)

2 tablespoons salsa or tomato paste

1 teaspoon chili powder

¼ teaspoon onion powder

¼ teaspoon dried oregano

¼ teaspoon ground cumin

¼ teaspoon garlic powder

¼ teaspoon sea salt

Pinch of cayenne pepper, or more to taste

2 cups cooked brown rice or quinoa

1 cup chopped tomatoes

1 cup chopped lettuce

¼ cup low-fat plain Greek yogurt

¼ cup grated sharp cheddar cheese

Heat the blend, salsa, and all of the spices in a small pot over medium-low heat, and stir to combine. Heat until just warmed through. Place ½ cup of rice in each bowl and top with ½ cup of the bean mixture. Divide the tomatoes, lettuce, yogurt, and cheese equally among them and serve.

Nutrition facts (per serving): 200 calories; 3 g fat; 86 mg sodium; 36 g carbs; 5 g fiber; 4 g sugar; 9 g protein

MISO-GINGER COD IN PARCHMENT

Makes 4 servings • Serving size: 1 parchment packet

This meal is great for company. There's something special about the parchment packets: Everyone gets their own little "present." The fish and veggies steam right inside and there are no pans to clean up. Just toss the parchment when you're done. Be careful when opening them, because you'll get a big whoosh of steam.

½ cup Miso-Ginger Dressing
(page 181)

Juice of 1 orange

1 bunch of large asparagus
spears, tough ends removed
(about 2 pounds)

1 pound snow peas

4 4-ounce cod fillets (about 1
pound total)

Sea salt and freshly ground
black pepper

Preheat the oven to 425 degrees. In a medium bowl, whisk together the dressing and orange juice. Lay 4 large sheets of parchment paper on a work surface. Place one quarter of the asparagus and snow peas on one end of each sheet of paper and top each portion of vegetables with a piece of fish. Drizzle one quarter of the dressing over each piece of fish and season with salt and pepper. Fold the other side of the parchment over the fish and veggies and, beginning at one end, fold in the edges of the parchment to seal it completely into a semicircular packet. Repeat with the remaining packets. Place the packets on a baking sheet and bake for 12 to 14 minutes, until the fish is just cooked through. Remove to plates and serve in the parchment (be careful opening them).

Nutrition facts (per serving): **205 calories; 2 g fat; 317 mg sodium; 15 g carbs; 6 g fiber; 3 g sugar; 31 g protein**

CITRUS-HERB ROASTED TURKEY WITH MUSHROOM GRAVY

Makes 4 servings • Serving size: 4 ounces turkey, about ¹/₂ cup mushrooms, plus ¹/₄ cup sauce

I'm kind of obsessed with this recipe; it's like a Thanksgiving meal you can make any day, thanks to quick-cooking turkey cutlets. And who could ever imagine that gravy could be healthy, but it is, thanks to White Bean Base Blend, loads of meaty-tasting mushrooms, and fresh rosemary. All the produce makes it a one-pan meal, too.

For the gravy

1 tablespoon extra-virgin olive oil

1 cup low-sodium chicken broth (or Bone Broth, page 56), divided

1 pound cremini mushrooms, chopped

½ teaspoon Worcestershire sauce

½ teaspoon onion powder

¼ teaspoon sea salt

2 tablespoons **White Bean Base Blend** (page 83)

2 teaspoons chopped fresh rosemary

For the turkey

1 tablespoon extra-virgin olive oil

1 pound turkey cutlets

Sea salt and freshly ground black pepper

½ lemon

Make the gravy: Heat the oil and 2 tablespoons of the broth over medium heat. Add the mushrooms and sauté for 8 to 10 minutes, until browned. Leave 1/2 cup of the mushrooms in the skillet and transfer the rest to a small bowl. Add the remaining broth, the Worcestershire sauce, onion powder, salt, the blend, and the rosemary to the skillet and simmer for 5 minutes. Carefully pour the gravy mixture into a high-powered blender and puree until smooth.

Meanwhile, prepare the turkey: Heat the oil in a skillet over medium-high heat. Cook the turkey for 3 to 5 minutes a side, until browned and cooked through. Toss the reserved mushrooms back into the pan with the turkey just before serving to rewarm them. Squeeze the juice from the lemon over the turkey and season with salt and pepper to taste. Divide among plates and pour the sauce over.

Nutrition facts (per serving): 219 calories; 8 g fat; 255 mg sodium; 6 g carbs; 4 g fiber; 1 g sugar; 29 g protein

PESTO PASTA WITH ROASTED SHRIMP

Makes 4 servings • Serving size: About 2 cups

I use pistachios in place of pine nuts for a modern spin on traditional pesto, and use Broccoli-Pea-Spinach Base Blend in the pesto to add volume, while cutting back on the usual amounts of oil and Parm. I personally find pistachios tastier, but (bonus!) they also happen to have double the protein, 20 percent fewer calories, and more fiber than pine nuts. And they're a lot more wallet friendly. Add shrimp and pasta and—heaven.

1 pound wild shrimp, peeled and deveined

½ tablespoon extra-virgin olive oil

Sea salt and freshly ground black pepper

6 ounces dry (or 3 cups cooked) whole grain linguine (or any other shape)

½ cup Pistachio Power Pesto (page 190)

Chopped fresh basil leaves, for garnish

Preheat the oven to 400 degrees. Toss the shrimp with the oil, season with salt and pepper, and spread in one layer on a baking sheet. Roast for 8 to 10 minutes until just pink and cooked through. Meanwhile, cook the pasta according to package directions. Toss the shrimp with the pasta and pesto. Garnish with basil and serve.

Nutrition facts (per serving): 339 calories; 10 g fat; 235 mg sodium; 31 g carbs; 6 g fiber; 2 g sugar; 31 g protein

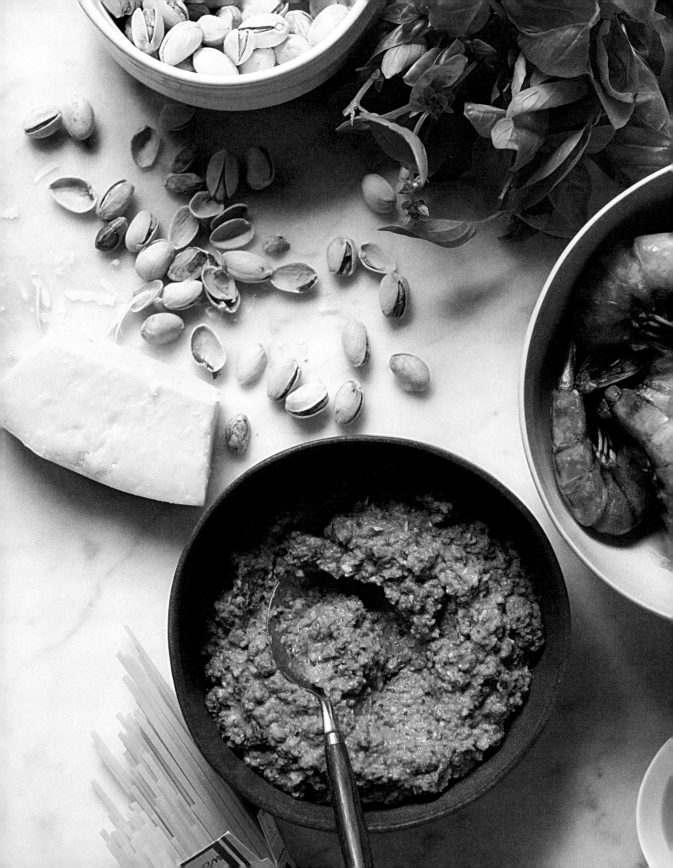

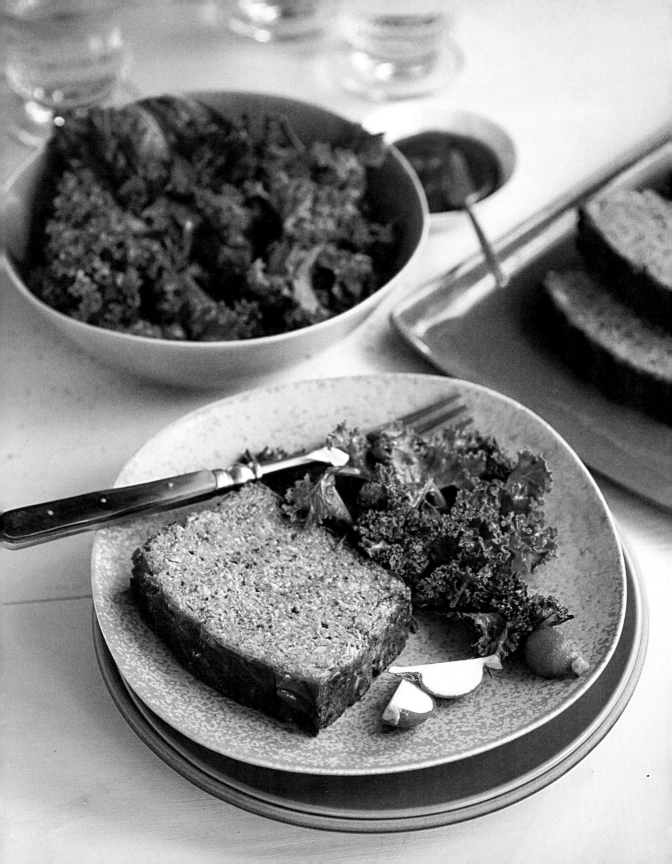

NOT YOUR MOM'S (TURKEY) MEAT LOAF

Makes 6 servings • Serving size: 1 1¹/₂-inch-thick slice, plus sautéed kale

Instead of the refined, nutrient-devoid white bread crumbs found in Aunt May's meat loaf, this recipe uses oats and flaxseed, which deliver a nice dose of fiber, antioxidants, and omega-3s. And the Black Bean–Blueberry–Baby Kale Base Blend gives this meat loaf incredible moisture, adds another hit of nutrition, and allows you to use half as much meat as most recipes.

For the meat loaf

½ cup **Black Bean–Blueberry–Baby Kale Base Blend** (page 100)

¼ teaspoon sea salt

Freshly ground black pepper

¼ teaspoon onion powder

1 large egg

1 teaspoon Worcestershire sauce

2 tablespoons ground flaxseed

½ cup oats, finely ground

1 tablespoon tomato paste

½ teaspoon dried oregano

1 pound lean ground turkey breast

Nonstick cooking spray

3 tablespoons organic ketchup (optional)

For the kale

1 tablespoon extra-virgin olive oil

1 11-ounce bag baby kale

Sea salt and freshly ground black pepper

Make the meat loaf: Preheat the oven to 350 degrees. In a large bowl, combine the first 10 ingredients and mix well with the back of a fork. Add the turkey and mix into the seasonings. Transfer to a standard-size loaf pan that's been misted with cooking spray and top with the ketchup, if using. Bake for 35 to 45 minutes, or until the meat reaches an internal temperature of 160 degrees.

Meanwhile, make the kale: Heat the oil in a skillet over medium heat. Add the kale and cover the pan for a few minutes to allow it to wilt down. Remove the lid and sauté until totally wilted and any liquid in the pan has cooked off. Season with salt and pepper to taste and serve with the meat loaf.

Nutrition facts (per serving): **227** calories; **10 g** fat; **271 mg** sodium; **16 g** carbs; **4 g** fiber; **1 g** sugar; **20 g** protein

MEATY MUSHROOM BOLOGNESE

Makes 6 servings • Serving size: 1 cup pasta, plus ¹/₂ cup sauce

The mushrooms in this dish allow you to use one third of the meat you'd usually use thanks to their natural meaty texture and flavor. Mushrooms are also nutrition powerhouses that boost your immunity, metabolism, and levels of vitamins D and B. And the Carrot–Sweet Potato Base Blend melds seamlessly into the sauce, while upping your antioxidant intake even more.

2 tablespoons extra-virgin olive oil

1 medium Vidalia onion, diced

1 to 2 garlic cloves, minced

½ pound 93% lean ground grass-fed beef (or turkey)

10 cremini mushrooms (about 10 ounces), diced

1 28-ounce box whole peeled tomatoes, with juice

½ teaspoon dried oregano

A few fresh basil leaves, torn

½ cup **Carrot–Sweet Potato Base Blend** (page 86)

¼ teaspoon sea salt

Freshly ground black pepper

Pinch of ground cinnamon

12 ounces whole grain rigatoni

⅓ cup freshly grated Parmesan cheese

Place a large skillet over medium heat. Add the oil and sauté the onion and garlic for 3 to 5 minutes. Stir in the turkey and mushrooms and cook for 5 to 8 minutes until brown, breaking up the meat with a wooden spoon. Crush the tomatoes with your hands and add them to the pan with the juices from the container. Add the oregano, basil, blend, salt, pepper to taste, and cinnamon and bring to a boil. Reduce the heat and simmer until the liquid is reduced by half, about 20 minutes.

Meanwhile, cook the pasta according to the package directions. Toss the sauce with the pasta and sprinkle with the Parmesan. Season with salt and pepper to taste and serve.

Nutrition facts (per serving): **348 calories; 10 g fat; 203 mg sodium; 47 g carbs; 7 g fiber; 3 g sugar; 19 g protein**

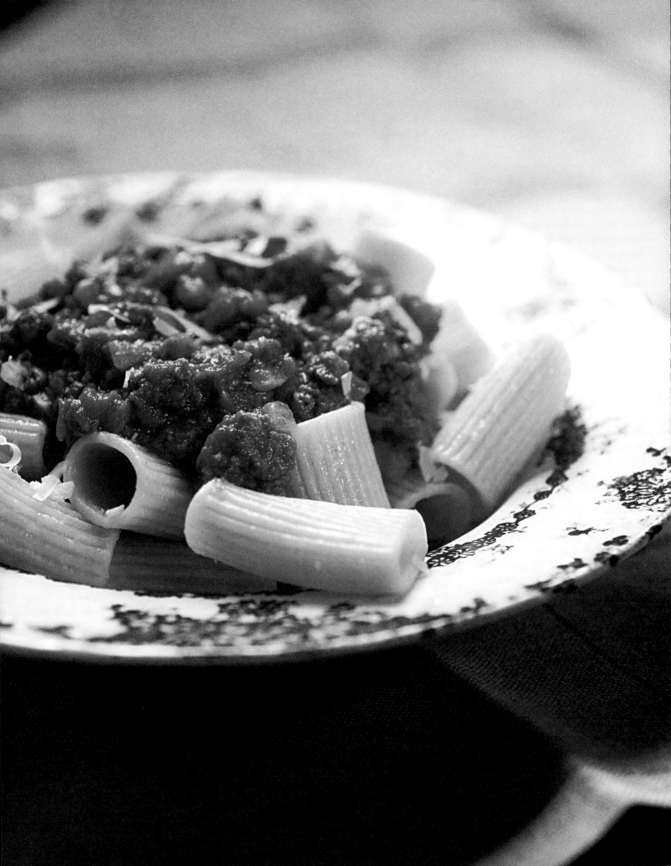

CRUNCHY TOFU STICKS WITH SMALL-BATCH KETCHUP

Makes 4 servings • Serving size: 4 to 5 sticks, plus 2 tablespoons ketchup

This is the perfect Meatless Monday meal. Don't pass it by because you don't love the texture of tofu. The tofu here is "meaty" and crunchy and not what you imagine typical tofu to be. I recommend pressing the tofu first: Just place the whole block between paper towels and put a weight on top of it (such as a foil-covered brick or this book). Let it sit in the fridge for at least 30 minutes and up to 2 days to get rid of some of the moisture. Don't skip the ketchup, either. The regular kind is surprisingly high in sugar and salt; this one's low on both and the Carrot–Sweet Potato Base Blend gives it even more nutrition.

For the tofu
½ cup almond meal*

¼ cup finely grated Parmesan cheese

¼ teaspoon sea salt

¼ teaspoon onion powder

½ teaspoon dried oregano

A few turns of freshly ground black pepper

1 ½ blocks (21 ounces) extra-firm tofu, cut horizontally, then cut into 18 sticks

Nonstick cooking spray

For the small-batch ketchup
2 tablespoons tomato paste

⅓ cup **Carrot–Sweet Potato Base Blend** (page 86)

1 teaspoon paprika

2 tablespoons balsamic vinegar

1 teaspoon raw honey

1 teaspoon Worcestershire sauce

Prepare the tofu: Preheat the oven to 425 degrees. Place the first 6 ingredients in a resealable plastic bag and shake to mix. Slice the blocks of tofu in half, then cut each one into ½-inch sticks. Lightly mist a baking sheet with cooking spray. Place the tofu sticks on the baking sheet, then mist the sticks with cooking spray. Bake for 10 minutes, then flip, mist the sticks again, and bake for 10 minutes more, until golden brown.

Meanwhile, make the ketchup: in a medium bowl, whisk together all of the ingredients.

Serve the tofu sticks hot with 2 tablespoons of the ketchup on the side of each portion.

* If you can't find almond meal at the store, it's easy to make. Soak raw almonds (with the skins still on) overnight, then drain, dry, and pulse them in a food processor until they form a meal-like consistency.

{ *Nutrition facts (per serving)*: 301 calories; 17 g fat; 224 mg sodium; 11 g carbs; 3 g fiber; 4 g sugar; 27 g protein }

MISO-KALE NOODLE BOWL

Makes 4 servings • Serving size: 2 cups

GF
V
DF

Noodle bowls sound healthy, but they're usually loaded with simple carb-y noodles and salt. This version is easy on the sodium and uses brown rice noodles to drastically lighten the entire dish. Grab your chopsticks.

3 cups water

3 tablespoons white miso paste, whisked into a little hot water to dissolve

1 cup **Chickpea-Zucchini Base Blend** (page 82)

1 cup firm tofu, cubed

2 cups chopped baby kale

4 ounces dried brown rice noodles

Seaweed sheets (optional)

Heat the water in a large pot over medium heat (not quite to a boil). Whisk in the miso and the blend. Add the tofu, kale, rice noodles, and seaweed sheets, if using, and cook for 2 minutes, or until the noodles are al dente. Serve.

{ *Nutrition facts (per serving)*: 238 calories; 5 g fat; 202 mg sodium; 39 g carbs; 6 g fiber; 3 g sugar; 12 g protein }

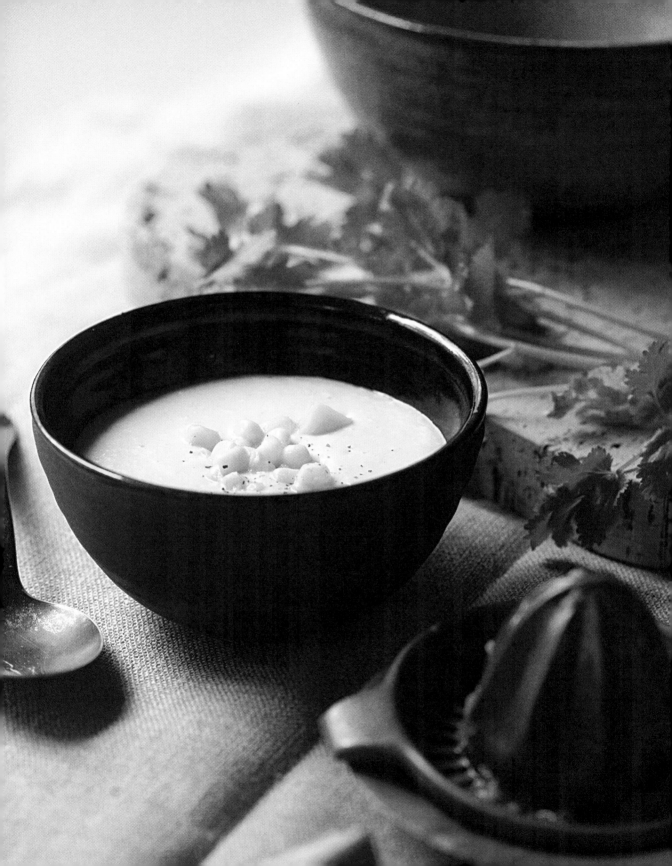

COCONUT CORN CHOWDER WITH CILANTRO AND LIME

Makes 4 servings • Serving size: 2 cups

I love chowder—it's such a comfort food—but I could never find a healthier version that was still just as satisfying. Until I created this dish. The Cauliflower Base Blend adds creaminess but saves you a whopping 205 calories and 14 grams of saturated fat per serving over using heavy cream.

1 tablespoon extra-virgin olive oil

1 medium Vidalia onion, diced

1 small new potato, diced (skin on)

¼ teaspoon sea salt

1 cup light coconut milk

2 cups low-sodium vegetable broth (or chicken broth)

1 cup **Cauliflower Base Blend** (page 84)

2 cups frozen or fresh corn kernels, ideally organic

Juice of 1 lime

Freshly ground black pepper

2 tablespoons chopped fresh cilantro

Heat the oil in a large soup pot over medium heat. Add the onion and sauté until slightly translucent, about 10 minutes. Add the potato and salt and cook for another 5 minutes. Stir in the coconut milk, broth, the blend, and the corn. Raise the heat and bring the soup to a boil, then reduce the heat and simmer for 20 minutes, or until the potatoes are tender. Transfer some of the soup to a high-powered blender and puree until smooth; carefully pour it back into the pot. Add more or less soup depending on how thick and chunky you like your chowder. (You can also use an immersion blender.) Stir in the lime juice just before serving and season with pepper. Top each bowl with cilantro and serve.

Nutrition facts (per serving): 204 calories; 8 g fat; 202 mg sodium; 31 g carbs; 3 g fiber; 10 g sugar; 6 g protein

* (if using vegetable broth)

CURRIED CHICKEN SALAD-STUFFED PITAS

Makes 4 servings • Serving size: ¹/₂ pita stuffed with 1 ¹/₄ cups chicken salad and ¹/₄ cup cucumber slices

White Bean Base Blend and yogurt replace the high-cal mayo used in traditional chicken salad. I love the exotic curry powder here; but if you don't care for it, you can leave it out. For an even quicker meal, pick up a store-bought rotisserie chicken.

¼ cup **White Bean Base Blend** (page 83)

⅓ cup plain low-fat Greek yogurt

Juice of ½ lemon

½ teaspoon Dijon mustard

1 to 2 teaspoons curry powder

Sea salt and freshly ground black pepper

3 cups chopped, cooked chicken breast

1 cup peeled and diced apple

2 whole grain pitas, halved

1 cup sliced cucumber

In a large bowl, whisk together the blend, yogurt, lemon juice, mustard, and curry powder. Season with sea salt and pepper to taste. Add the chicken and apple and toss to combine. Divide the chicken salad among the pita halves, stuff each with cucumber slices, and serve.

Nutrition facts (per serving): 274 calories; 5 g fat; 159 mg sodium; 20 g carbs; 5 g fiber; 7 g sugar; 38 g protein

(NOT) FORBIDDEN RICE SALAD WITH RASPBERRY-BEET VINAIGRETTE

GF
V

Makes 4 servings • Serving size: 1 1/2 cups salad, plus 1/2 cup rice

The pigment that gives black rice its color contains more antioxidants than blueberries—and it's far more nutritious than brown rice. I love the chewiness of it, too. The blend in this recipe (Raspberry-Beet) comes from the easy-to-make vinaigrette.

⅔ cup black or wild rice

½ cup **Raspberry-Beet Vinaigrette** (page 187)

4 cups baby spinach

¼ cup chopped walnuts

¼ cup fresh raspberries (or dried no-sugar-added cranberries)

¼ cup crumbled feta cheese

Sea salt and freshly ground black pepper

Cook the rice according to the package directions and set aside to cool. Toss the rice with ¼ cup of the vinaigrette. In a large bowl, toss together the spinach, walnuts, and raspberries. Put 1 ½ cups of salad on each plate, top with 1 tablespoon goat cheese, and drizzle with the remaining dressing. Add ½ cup rice to each salad. Season with salt and pepper to taste and serve.

Nutrition facts (per serving): 287 calories; 15 g fat; 317 mg sodium; 36 g carbs; 6 g fiber; 6 g sugar; 8 g protein

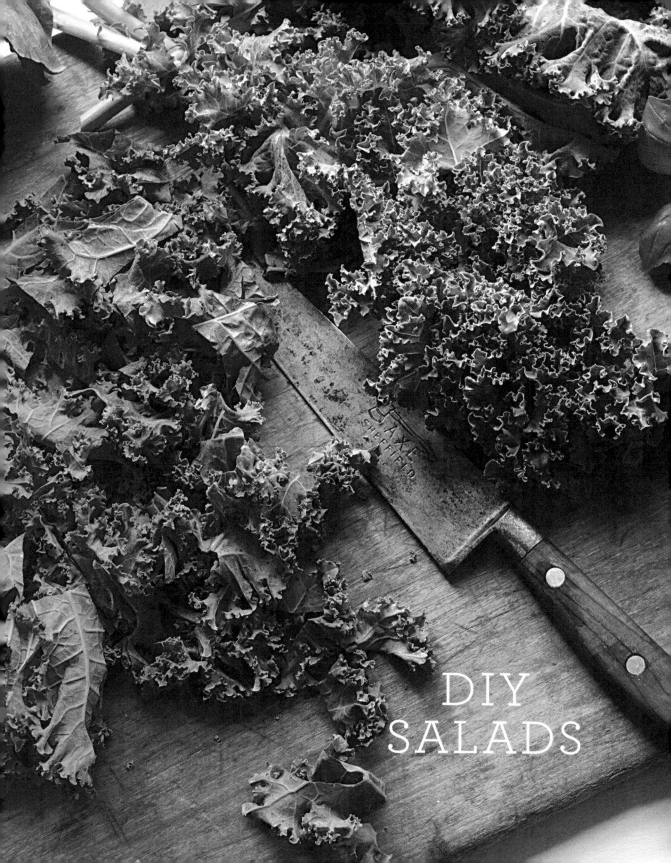

DIY
SALADS

Each of these dressings uses my blends to cut calories; and each adds enough nutrition that you don't need to eat your weight in greens to get your daily allowance. I've given a simple salad suggestion to pair with each dressing, but you'll find other recipes in the book that use these dressings, too. You can also keep a batch of dressing in the fridge and add a serving to whatever mix of greens you've got in your fridge—ideal for a last-minute lunch or dinner. The blend in each dressing injects a broader array of phytonutrients into your salad, so you can keep the rest of the meal simple.

MISO-GINGER DRESSING

Makes 4 servings • Serving size: 2 tablespoons

GF
LC
V
DF

1 rounded tablespoon white or yellow miso paste

2 tablespoons boiling water

⅓ cup **Carrot-Sweet Potato Base Blend** (page 86)

1-inch piece peeled fresh ginger, grated (about 1 tablespoon), or ¼ teaspoon ground ginger

2 tablespoons rice vinegar

½ teaspoon sesame oil

1 tablespoon peanut or grapeseed oil

Whisk the miso paste and water together in a small heatproof bowl, then whisk in all of the other ingredients.

Nutrition facts (per serving): 32 calories; 5 g fat; 227 mg sodium; 5 g carbs; 1 g fiber; 1 g sugar; 1 g protein

— TRY IT ON —

Warm Wilted Baby Bok Choy Salad (serves 4)

GF
V
DF

Slice 2 baby bok choy in half lengthwise (about 6 cups total) and sauté in 1 tablespoon olive oil just until wilted. Place ½ cup cooked brown rice on each of 4 plates and divide the bok choy among them. Pour 2 tablespoons dressing over each salad and serve.

Nutrition facts (per serving): 180 calories; 5 g fat; 277 mg sodium; 29 g carbs; 4 g fiber; 3 g sugar; 4 g protein

ALL HAIL EGGLESS CAESAR DRESSING

Makes 4 servings • Serving size: 2 tablespoons

2 tablespoons white or red wine vinegar

2 tablespoons freshly squeezed lemon juice

6 tablespoons **Cauliflower Base Blend** (page 84)

½ teaspoon Worcestershire sauce

1 to 2 small garlic cloves

3 to 4 anchovy fillets

2 tablespoons extra-virgin olive oil

1 tablespoon freshly grated Parmesan cheese

Puree the first 6 ingredients until smooth. Turn the blender on low and slowly drizzle the olive oil through the feed tube, then pulse in the Parmesan cheese.

Nutrition facts (per serving): **74 calories; 7 g fat; 153 mg sodium; 2 g carbs; 0 g fiber; 1 g sugar; 1 g protein**

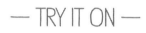

— TRY IT ON —

Gold Ribbon Kale Caesar Salad (serves 4)

Remove and discard the stems from 1 bunch of kale (about 1 pound) and cut the leaves into ribbons. In a large bowl, toss the kale with ½ cup dressing. Grate 4 hard-boiled eggs on top.

Nutrition facts (per serving): **217 calories; 13 g fat; 272 mg sodium; 16 g carbs; 3 g fiber; 1 g sugar; 12 g protein**

EVEN GREENER
GODDESS DRESSING

Makes 4 servings • Serving size: 2 tablespoons

¼ cup loosely packed fresh basil leaves, minced

Zest of 1 lemon plus 1 tablespoon freshly squeezed lemon juice

¼ cup **Sweet Pea Base Blend** (page 92)

2 tablespoons plain low-fat Greek yogurt

⅛ teaspoon sea salt

1 tablespoon chopped fresh chives

Whisk all of the ingredients together in a bowl until well combined.

Nutrition facts (per serving): **17 calories; 0 g fat; 34 mg sodium; 3 g carbs; 1 g fiber; 1 g sugar; 2 g protein**

— TRY IT ON —

Grilled Hearts of Romaine (serves 4)

Preheat an outdoor grill (or grill pan) to medium and brush the grill with oil. Rinse 4 whole hearts of romaine and pat dry. Cut each in half lengthwise so they're still held together by their cores, then lightly brush with 1 tablespoon oil. Grill for about 2 minutes, turning once to char each side slightly. Divide among 4 plates and drizzle each with 2 tablespoons of dressing.

Nutrition facts (per serving): **63 calories; 3 g fat; 42 mg sodium; 5 g carbs; 3 g fiber; 2 g sugar; 3 g protein**

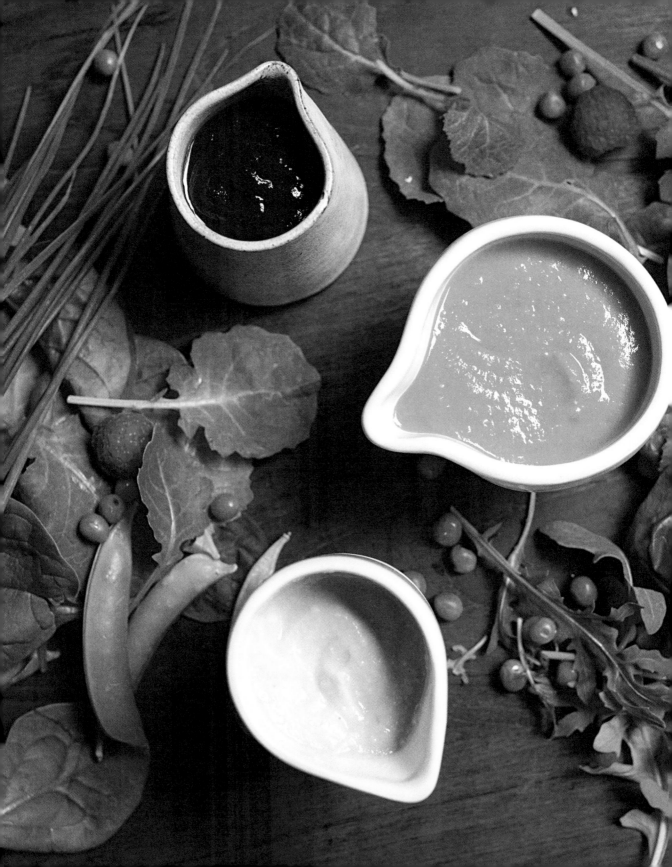

CREAMY FETA DRESSING

Makes 4 servings • Serving size: 2 tablespoons

½ cup peeled, sliced cucumber

Zest of 1 lemon, plus 1 ½ tablespoons freshly squeezed lemon juice

½ teaspoon dried oregano

3 tablespoons **Cauliflower Base Blend** (page 84)

1 tablespoon extra-virgin olive oil

2 tablespoons plain low-fat Greek yogurt

2 tablespoons crumbled feta cheese

Puree all of the ingredients until smooth.

Nutrition facts (per serving): 58 calories; 5 g fat; 43 mg sodium; 2 g carbs; 1 g fiber; 1 g sugar; 2 g protein

— TRY IT ON —

Greek-Style Chopped Salad (serves 4)

Chop 2 large tomatoes, 1 large seedless cucumber, and 1 seeded green bell pepper. Thinly slice ¼ cup red onion. Toss the veggies in a large bowl with ¼ cup pitted kalamata olives and ½ cup dressing and divide among plates. Sprinkle 1 ½ tablespoons feta over each salad and serve.

Nutrition facts (per serving): 175 calories; 12 g fat; 329 mg sodium; 12 g carbs; 2 g fiber; 6 g sugar; 8 g protein

REVAMPED RUSSIAN DRESSING

Makes 4 servings • *Serving size: 2 tablespoons*

1 ½ tablespoons tomato paste

¼ cup **White Bean Base Blend** (page 83)

2 tablespoons cider vinegar

1 ½ teaspoons raw honey

¼ teaspoon onion powder

1 tablespoon extra-virgin olive oil

1 tablespoon chopped pickles (or relish)

Sea salt and freshly ground black pepper

Puree the first 6 ingredients until smooth. Pulse in the pickles, if using, season with salt and pepper to taste and serve.

Nutrition facts (per serving): 66 calories; 4 g fat; 44 mg sodium; 8 g carbs; 1 g fiber; 3 g sugar; 2 g protein

— TRY IT ON —

Russian Slaw (serves 4)

In a large bowl, toss 1 14-ounce package coleslaw or broccoli slaw mix with ½ cup Russian dressing. Divide among 4 plates, season with salt and pepper to taste, and serve.

Nutrition facts (per serving): 92 calories; 4 g fat; 64 mg sodium; 14 g carbs; 4 g fiber; 7 g sugar; 3 g protein

RASPBERRY-BEET VINAIGRETTE

Makes 4 servings • Serving size: 2 tablespoons

GF LC V DF

¼ cup **Raspberry-Beet Base Blend** (page 94)

2 tablespoons extra-virgin olive oil

2 tablespoons balsamic vinegar

Sea salt

1 teaspoon raw honey

Whisk all of the ingredients together in a small bowl.

Nutrition facts (per serving): 76 calories; 7 g fat; 6 mg sodium; 5 g carbs; 1 g fiber; 4 g sugar; 0 g protein

— TRY IT ON —

Goat Cheese and Arugula Salad (serves 4)

GF LC V

Divide 8 cups of arugula among 4 plates. Sprinkle each with 1 tablespoon chopped walnuts and 1 tablespoon goat cheese and drizzle with 2 tablespoons dressing. Season with salt and pepper to taste and serve.

Nutrition facts (per serving): 158 calories; 14 g fat; 50 mg sodium; 7 g carbs; 2 g fiber; 5 g sugar; 4 g protein

DIY PASTA
DINNERS

Who doesn't love a comforting bowl of pasta? And you can have it—and feel good about it—because the blends in each of these pasta dishes add fiber and key nutrients while adding bulk to your meal, so you get to put more in that bowl. I've given serving suggestions for each of the sauces below, but feel free to experiment. They're super-versatile and could go over a piece of chicken or fish as easily as pasta—and I've included nutrition info, so you can use them in whatever way you'd like and still know your calories are in line. The sauces freeze really well, too, so any extras can be pulled out for a last-minute dinner.

CREAMY NO-TOMATO PASTA SAUCE

Makes 4 servings • Serving size: 1/2 cup

GF
LC
V

1 cup **Carrot–Sweet Potato Base Blend** (page 86)

½ cup low-sodium vegetable broth (or chicken broth)

1 tablespoon extra-virgin olive oil

Pinch of ground nutmeg

2 to 3 tablespoons low-fat milk or light coconut milk

Sea salt and freshly ground black pepper

Whisk the blend, broth, oil, nutmeg, and milk together in a medium pot over medium heat for 5 minutes, until warmed through. Season with salt and pepper to taste and serve.

Nutrition facts (per serving): **61 calories; 4 g fat; 41 mg sodium; 6 g carbs; 4 g fiber; 2 g sugar; 1 g protein**

— TRY IT ON —

Roasted Cod with Penne (serves 4)

Toss 1 cup warm sauce with 2 cups hot cooked and drained whole grain bucatini or spaghetti. Top with 8 ounces roasted cod, cut into pieces, and divide among 4 bowls. Season with salt and pepper to taste and serve.

Nutrition facts (per serving): **175 calories; 3 g fat; 67 mg sodium; 22 g carbs; 4 g fiber; 1 g sugar; 17 g protein**

PISTACHIO POWER PESTO

Makes 4 servings • Serving size: 2 tablespoons

GF LC V *

½ cup **Broccoli-Pea-Spinach Base Blend** (page 90)

2 cups loosely packed fresh basil leaves (about 40 leaves), plus a few for garnish

2 tablespoons freshly grated Parmesan cheese

2 tablespoons pistachio halves

1 to 2 garlic cloves

1 tablespoon extra-virgin olive oil

3 to 4 tablespoons low-sodium vegetable broth (or Bone Broth, page 56, or chicken broth)

Sea salt and freshly ground black pepper

Place the first 6 ingredients into a high-powered blender and pulse to combine; add broth to the mixture 1 tablespoon at a time and pulse to the desired pesto consistency. Season with salt and pepper to taste.

Note: Leftover pesto can be stored in the fridge for 3 days or frozen for up to 3 months. Add a thin film of oil to the top before storing to prevent the pesto from turning brown.

Nutrition facts (per serving): 69 calories; 6 g fat; 65 mg sodium; 4 g carbs; 1 g fiber; 1 g sugar; 2 g protein

— TRY IT ON —

Chicken with Bow Ties (serves 4)

Place ½ cup pesto into a large bowl with 8 ounces cooked, diced chicken. Add 2 cups hot cooked and drained whole grain bow tie pasta and divide among 4 bowls. Season with salt and pepper to taste and serve.

Nutrition facts (per serving): 250 calories; 8 g fat; 110 mg sodium; 22 g carbs; 4 g fiber; 1 g sugar; 24 g protein

* *(if made with vegetable broth)*

MAKE-IT-IN-MINUTES MARINARA SAUCE

Makes 12 servings • Serving size: ¹/₂ cup

GF LC V DF

2 tablespoons extra-virgin olive oil

1 garlic clove, finely minced

1 sweet onion, finely chopped or pureed (about 1 cup)

½ cup **Carrot–Sweet Potato Base Blend** (page 86)

A few fresh basil leaves, or ¼ teaspoon dried basil

¼ teaspoon dried oregano

1 28-ounce box whole peeled tomatoes, with juice

¼ teaspoon sea salt

A few turns of freshly ground black pepper

Heat the oil in a large skillet over medium heat. Add the garlic and onion and sauté until they are slightly translucent, but not brown, stirring occasionally, 6 to 8 minutes. Add the blend, basil, and oregano. Crush the tomatoes with your hands to break them up, add them to the skillet with their juices, and bring to a boil. Reduce the heat and simmer, uncovered, for 15 to 20 minutes, until the sauce thickens. Season with salt and pepper to taste. (If you want smoother sauce, transfer it to a blender and puree in batches.) Use immediately or store in the refrigerator for up to 1 week, or freezer for up to 6 months.

Nutrition facts (per serving): **46 calories; 2 g fat; 66 mg sodium; 5 g carbs; 1 g fiber; 3 g sugar; 1 g protein**

— TRY IT ON —

Hearty Turkey Spaghetti (serves 4)

Brown 8 ounces lean ground turkey in 1 tablespoon olive oil. Toss the browned turkey with 1 cup warm sauce and 2 cups hot, cooked and drained whole grain spaghetti and divide among 4 bowls. Season with salt and pepper to taste and serve.

Nutrition facts (per serving): **259 calories; 8 g fat; 138 mg sodium; 27 g carbs; 5 g fiber; 5 g sugar; 18 g protein**

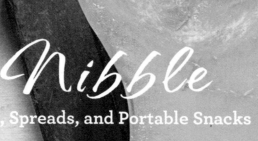

Nibble

Dips, Spreads, and Portable Snacks

Each of these snacks is designed to be like a mini meal and contain a good mix of protein, healthy fat, and fiber—not like the high-carb snacks that people usually eat between meals, like chips. They'll keep your blood sugar stable, prevent cravings (and a mean case of the hangries), and get you out of the mindset that snacks are something that come out of a package. And research shows that people who eat 5 or 6 times a day weigh less and have smaller waistlines than those who skip snacks or eat less frequently.

I've made prepping snacks even simpler by listing the blend that each one uses in the chart below so you can choose a recipe based on whichever ones you have in your fridge. I've also noted where you can sub in another blend for the one I call for in the recipe. Many of them are totally interchangeable.

THE DISH	THE BASE BLEND
Gingered Squash Blend	Butternut Squash–Apple Base Blend (or any Orange Base Blend)
Bean and Goat Cheese Blend	Chickpea-Zucchini Base Blend (or White Bean Base Blend)
Rosemary–White Bean Blend	White Bean Base Blend
Cauliflower-Chive Blend	Cauliflower Base Blend
Every-Day-Is-a-Holiday Sweet Potato Blend	Carrot–Sweet Potato Base Blend
Cauliflower Parmesan Biscuits	Cauliflower Base Blend (or any White Base Blend)
Kale Chips with Sour Cream and Onion Dip	Cauliflower Base Blend
Creamy Kale Guac	Sweet Pea–Baby Kale Base Blend (or any Green Base Blend)
Curried Deviled Eggs	Chickpea-Zucchini Base Blend (or White Bean Base Blend)
4 P.M. Protein Cookie	White Bean Base Blend (or Chickpea-Zucchini Base Blend)

THE DISH	THE BASE BLEND
Crab and Artichoke Dip	White Bean Base Blend (or any White Base Blend)
Artichoke–Kalamata Olive Hummus	Chickpea-Zucchini Base Blend (or White Bean Base Blend)
Roasted Red Pepper Hummus	Cauliflower Base Blend (or any White Base Blend)
Jumping Bean Dip	Black Bean–Blueberry–Baby Kale Base Blend
Lentil-Carrot Curry Dip	Carrot–Sweet Potato Base Blend
Creamy White Bean "Butter" Dip	White Bean Base Blend (or Chickpea-Zucchini Base Blend)
Coffee-Chia Brewsicles	Blueberry–Baby Spinach Base Blend (or Mixed Berry–Baby Kale Base Blend)

1-MINUTE SNACKS

Here's the idea behind these: Start with a Base Blend, add a few other simple ingredients, and voilà! You have a tasty, super-healthy snack in seconds.

GINGERED SQUASH BLEND

• Makes 1 serving •

½ cup **Butternut Squash–Apple Base Blend** (page 87)

½ tablespoon pure maple syrup

¼ teaspoon grated peeled fresh ginger, or a pinch of ground ginger

Pinch of sea salt

Warm all of the ingredients in a small saucepan over medium-low heat, mixing well to combine, and serve.

Nutrition facts: 82 calories; 0 g fat; 2 mg sodium; 20 g carbs; 2 g fiber; 15 g sugar; 1 g protein

BEAN AND GOAT CHEESE BLEND

½ cup **Chickpea-Zucchini Base Blend** (page 82)

A few finely minced fresh basil leaves

Pinch of sea salt

1 tablespoon crumbled goat cheese

Warm all of the ingredients except the goat cheese in a small saucepan over medium-low heat, mixing well to combine. Serve with the goat cheese crumbled on top.

Nutrition facts: 115 calories; 3 g fat; 250 mg sodium; 17 g carbs; 5 g fiber; 3 g sugar; 6 g protein

ROSEMARY–WHITE BEAN BLEND

¼ cup **White Bean Base Blend** (page 83)

1 teaspoon extra-virgin olive oil

⅛ teaspoon minced fresh rosemary or

thyme

Pinch of red pepper flakes

Pinch of sea salt

Warm all of the ingredients in a small saucepan over medium-low heat, mixing well to combine, and serve.

Nutrition facts: 139 calories; 8 g fat; 31 mg sodium; 13 g carbs; 4 g fiber; 0 g sugar; 5 g protein

CAULIFLOWER-CHIVE BLEND

• Makes 1 serving •

1 cup **Cauliflower Base Blend** (page 84)

½ tablespoon extra-virgin olive oil

2 tablespoons low-sodium vegetable broth

or low-fat milk

Handful of chopped fresh chives

Pinch of sea salt

Warm all of the ingredients in a small saucepan over medium-low heat, mixing well to combine, and serve.

Nutrition facts: 105 calories; 7 g fat; 60 mg sodium; 9 g carbs; 4 g fiber; 4 g sugar; 4 g protein

* *(if using broth)*

EVERY-DAY-IS-A-HOLIDAY SWEET POTATO BLEND

Makes 4 servings • Serving size: 2/3 cup

2 cups **Carrot–Sweet Potato Base Blend** (page 86)

2 tablespoons pure maple syrup

½ cup unsweetened almond or coconut

milk

¼ teaspoon sea salt

¼ teaspoon ground cinnamon

Warm all of the ingredients in a medium pot, mixing well to combine, and serve.

Nutrition facts (per serving): 76 calories; 1 g fat; 214 mg sodium; 18 g carbs; 3 g fiber; 10 g sugar; 1 g protein

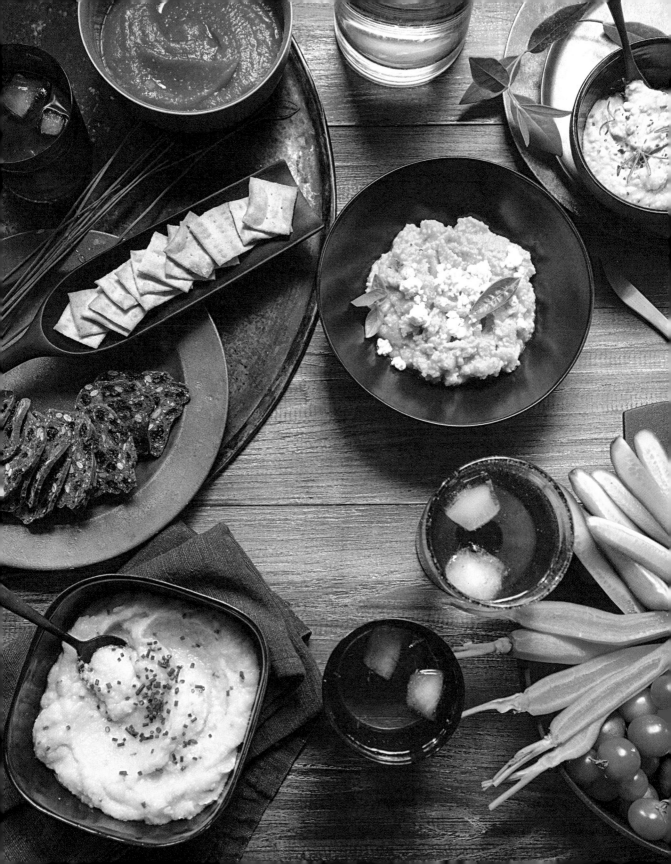

SMOKED SALMON SPREAD WITH CAPERS AND CHIVES

Makes 3 servings • Serving size: 2 tablespoons

This recipe doesn't use one of the Base Blends, but it does have pureed cucumber. Start straining the Greek yogurt before you do anything else so it'll be ready by the time the rest of the ingredients are put together. Serve this spread on a large whole grain cracker or half of a scooped-out whole wheat bagel for a satisfying snack that comes in under 150 calories.

2 tablespoons DIY Cream Cheese (page 128)

2 tablespoons pureed cucumber (from about ⅓ small peeled, seeded, and chopped cucumber)

1 teaspoon capers, drained

1 teaspoon chopped fresh chives

Squeeze of fresh lemon juice

½ ounce smoked salmon, chopped

Stir all of the ingredients together in a small bowl and serve.

Nutrition facts (per serving): 26 calories; 1 g fat; 46 mg sodium; 2 g carbs; 0 g fiber; 1 g sugar; 3 g protein

CAULIFLOWER PARMESAN BISCUITS

Makes 6 servings • Serving size: 1 biscuit

Biscuits are normally carb and fat bombs, but these have less than half the calories and carbs. And you also get cancer-fighting cruciferous veggies in this one. If you can't find white whole wheat flour, do a 50-50 mix of all-purpose flour and whole wheat flour.

Nonstick cooking spray

½ cup white whole wheat flour

¼ teaspoon sea salt

½ tablespoon baking powder

3 tablespoons extra-virgin olive oil

¼ cup low-fat milk

⅓ cup **Cauliflower Base Blend** (page 84)

3 tablespoons freshly grated Parmesan cheese

Preheat the oven to 400 degrees. Mist a baking sheet with nonstick cooking spray. In a large bowl, whisk together the flour, salt, and baking powder. Add the oil, milk, and the blend and mix well to combine. Drop heaping tablespoons of batter onto the baking sheet, leaving several inches in between. Top each biscuit with ½ tablespoon of the Parmesan and bake for about 15 minutes, until the biscuits are golden brown around the edges. Serve warm.

Nutrition facts (per serving): 106 calories; 7 g fat; 204 mg sodium; 8 g carbs; 1 g fiber; 0 g sugar; 3 g protein

GF LC V

KALE CHIPS WITH SOUR CREAM AND ONION DIP

Makes 8 servings • Serving size: 2 tablespoons dip and a handful of kale chips

As a kid, I loved to dunk potato chips in that junky dip you make with onion soup mix, and this is my way of replicating that delicious experience. I also added a bunch of spices to kick up the basic kale chip that everyone already knows and loves; I was going for a Doritos taste here. Delicious! Tip: Make sure the kale leaves are really dry when you put them in the oven, and don't overcrowd the pan, or they won't crisp up as well. I like lacinato (aka dinosaur) kale because its long, flat leaves are sturdy and turn out crunchy—but any type of kale will work here.

For the kale chips

¼ teaspoon garlic powder

½ teaspoon onion powder

1 teaspoon dried minced onions

⅛ teaspoon sea salt

6 cups lacinato kale leaves, washed, tough stems removed and patted dry

1 tablespoon extra-virgin olive oil

4 tablespoons freshly grated Parmesan cheese

For the dip

1 tablespoon extra-virgin olive oil

½ cup finely diced onion

3 tablespoons **Cauliflower Base Blend** (page 84)

½ cup low-fat Greek yogurt

¼ teaspoon onion powder

⅛ teaspoon sea salt

Freshly ground black pepper

Chopped fresh chives (optional)

Make the kale chips: Preheat the oven to 300 degrees. Mix the first 4 ingredients in a small bowl. Place the kale on a baking sheet in a single layer and toss with the olive oil. Massage the spice mixture into the kale, then evenly sprinkle the Parmesan on top. Bake for 30 minutes, flipping the kale once halfway through cooking, until the leaves are browned and crisp.

Meanwhile, make the dip: Heat the oil in a small skillet and sauté the onion over medium-low heat until lightly browned, about 10 minutes. Transfer the onion to a medium bowl and stir together the remaining ingredients for the dip.

Nutrition facts (per serving): 73 calories;
4 g fat; 118 mg sodium; 7 g carbs; 1 g fiber;
1 g sugar; 4 g protein

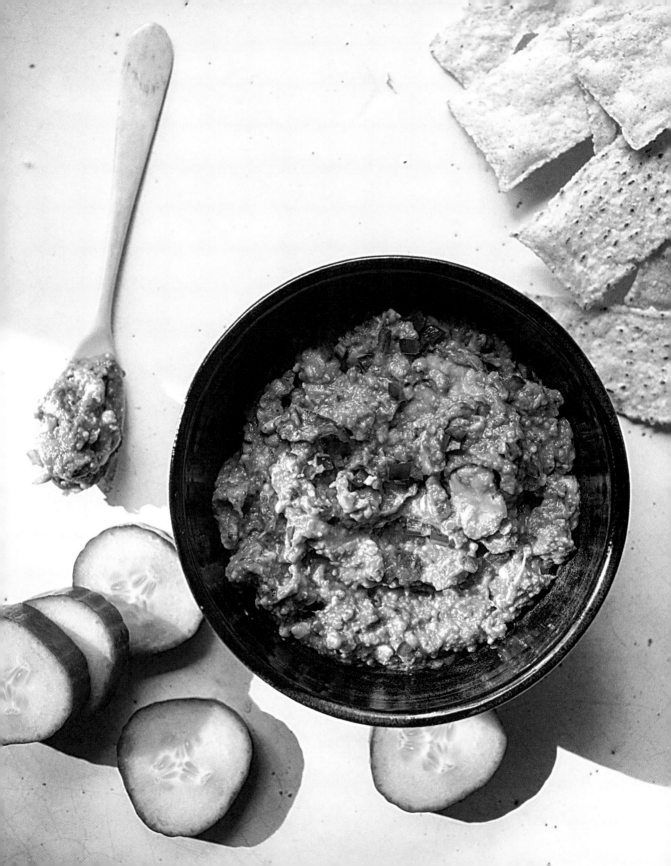

CREAMY KALE GUAC

Makes 16 servings • Serving size: 2 tablespoons

GF LC V DF

Guacamole is healthy in and of itself, but it's also one of those calorie-dense foods that can go from a snack to a meal pretty quickly. The blend in this version extends the volume of the dish by 50 percent, while taking down the calories. Serve the guac with cucumber rounds or strips of red or yellow bell pepper for dipping.

2 ripe Hass avocados

½ cup **Sweet Pea–Baby Kale Base Blend** (page 91)

Juice of 1 lime

2 tablespoons finely chopped fresh basil leaves

¼ teaspoon sea salt

A few turns of freshly ground black pepper

½ cup minced red onion (optional)

1 small jalapeño, seeded and minced (optional)

Halve the avocados lengthwise, remove the pit, and scoop the flesh into a small bowl. Add the remaining ingredients, mixing lightly with a fork and serve.

Nutrition facts (per serving): 42 calories; 3 g fat; 46 mg sodium; 4 g carbs; 2 g fiber; 1 g sugar; 1 g protein

CURRIED DEVILED EGGS

Makes 6 servings • Serving size: 2 deviled egg halves

I use Chickpea-Zucchini Base Blend as a stand-in for the mayo in this recipe. It lends a creamy hummus-like texture that makes the eggs healthier and lighter—with half the calories of the standard sat-fat-laden version. If you're not a curry fan, leave it out; they'll taste just as yummy without it.

6 large hard-boiled eggs, peeled

¾ cup **Chickpea-Zucchini Base Blend** (page 82)

¼ teaspoon sea salt

Freshly ground black pepper

¼ teaspoon curry powder

½ teaspoon Dijon mustard

½ teaspoon paprika

Slice the eggs lengthwise, pop out the yolks, and place 3 of them in a medium bowl. (Reserve or discard the remaining yolks.) Mash the blend, salt, pepper, curry powder, and mustard into the yolks and spoon—or pipe—the mixture back into the 12 egg white halves. Dust the tops with the paprika and serve.

Nutrition facts (per serving): 69 calories; 3 g fat; 218 mg sodium; 5 g carbs; 1 g fiber; 1 g sugar; 6 g protein

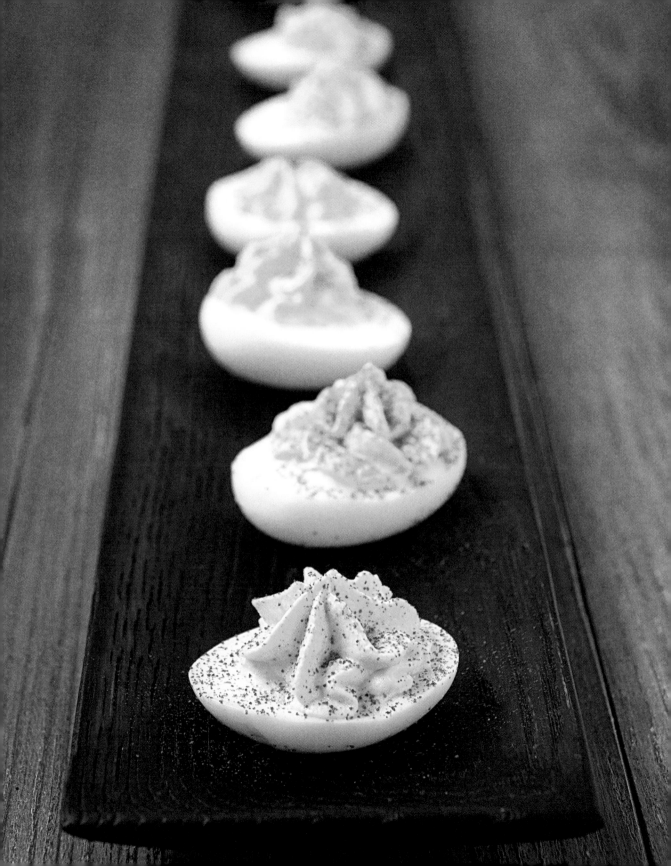

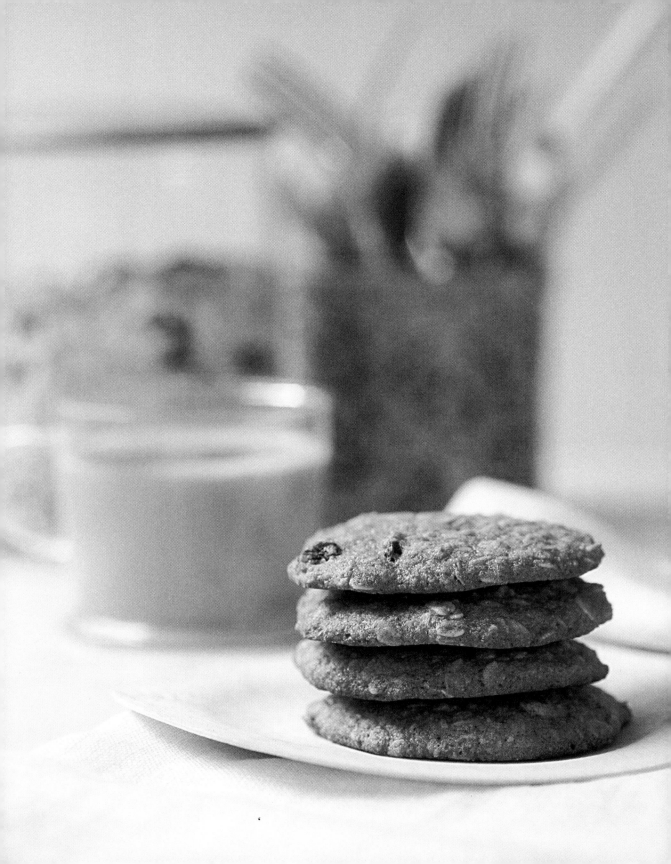

4 P.M. PROTEIN COOKIE

DF*

Makes 12 servings • Serving size: 1 cookie

The late afternoon is usually vending machine time—when we reach for pretzels or chips because our blood sugar (and willpower!) is low. Hello, simple carbs! But what you really need at a time like this is sustaining protein. Each oatmeal raisin cookie has as much protein as an egg.

5 tablespoons coconut oil

¼ cup **White Bean Base Blend** (page 83)

¼ cup pure maple syrup

1 large egg

½ teaspoon pure vanilla extract

⅓ cup vanilla protein powder

1 tablespoon ground flaxseed

½ teaspoon baking soda

½ teaspoon ground cinnamon

¼ teaspoon sea salt

1 ¼ cups rolled oats

½ cup whole wheat pastry flour

¼ cup raisins (optional)

Preheat the oven to 350 degrees. Line a baking sheet with parchment paper. In the bowl of an electric mixer fitted with a paddle attachment, cream the oil and the blend together on medium-high speed. Add the maple syrup, egg, and vanilla. Add the remaining ingredients and mix until combined. Place heaping tablespoons of batter on the baking sheet a few inches apart. Bake for 12 minutes, until the cookies are golden brown.

Nutrition facts (per serving): 141 calories; 7 g fat; 111 mg sodium; 16 g carbs; 2 g fiber; 4 g sugar; 5 g protein

* *(if using dairy-free protein powder)*

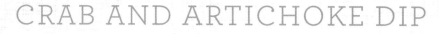

CRAB AND ARTICHOKE DIP

Makes 4 servings • Serving size: 2 tablespoons dip and 6 whole grain pita chips

This dip is so decadent you almost won't believe it doesn't have the cream cheese, sour cream, mayo, and tons of Parm that traditional versions have. It's important to use real Parmigiano-Reggiano cheese that has the official Italian D.O.P. seal (you'll see those letters on the rind). It's more expensive, but it tastes light-years better than the ordinary Parmesan you find at the store.

4 frozen or canned artichoke hearts, chopped

2 tablespoons **White Bean Base Blend** (page 83)

¼ cup plain low-fat Greek yogurt

½ tablespoon freshly squeezed lemon juice

3 tablespoons freshly grated Parmesan cheese, divided

4 ounces fresh lump crabmeat

Whole grain pita chips, for serving

Preheat the oven to 375 degrees. If using frozen artichokes, run them under cold water to slightly thaw; drain. In a large bowl, combine the artichokes, the blend, the yogurt, lemon juice, 1 tablespoon of the cheese, and the crabmeat. Transfer the mixture into an ovenproof ramekin and sprinkle the top with the remaining 2 tablespoons cheese. Bake for 10 to 12 minutes, until the top is bubbly and golden. Serve with whole grain pita chips.

Nutrition facts (per serving for the dip): 58 calories; 1 g fat; 328 mg sodium; 5 g carbs; 2 g fiber; 1 g sugar; 7 g protein

Nutrition facts (per serving for dip with chips): 129 calories; 4 g fat; 497 mg sodium; 14 g carbs; 3 g fiber; 1 g sugar; 10 g protein

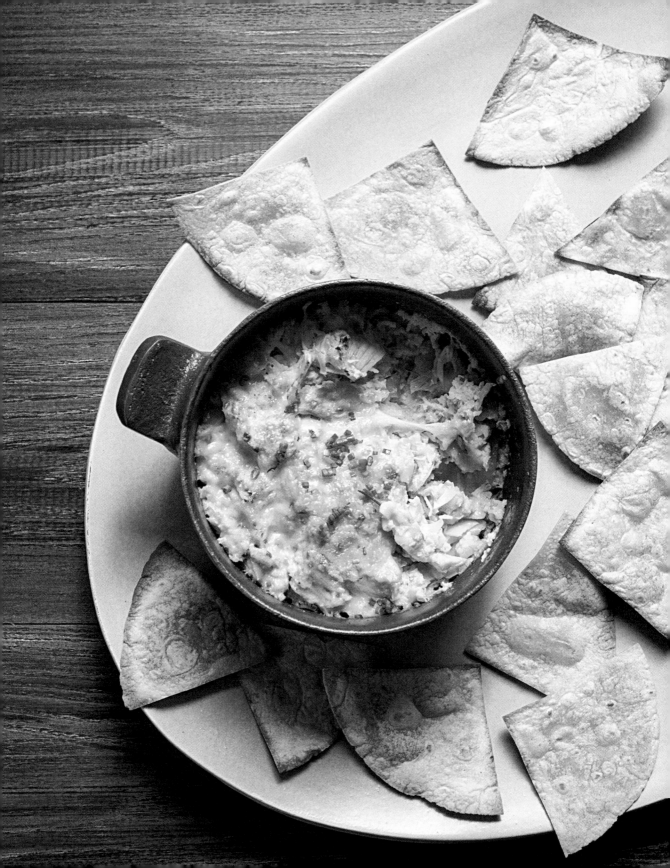

GF
LC
V
DF

ARTICHOKE-KALAMATA OLIVE HUMMUS

Makes 16 servings • Serving size: 2 tablespoons dip and 1 cup veggies

Hummus is everywhere these days: Supermarkets have entire walls of it, and you can even buy it at the gas station! So why bother to make your own? Because everything fresh tastes better, and this hummus only takes thirty seconds to put together. It also has more nutrient-rich veggies than the kind you'd buy and about half the calories.

1 teaspoon chia seeds, soaked in 3 tablespoons water for 10 minutes

1 cup **Chickpea-Zucchini Base Blend** (page 82) (or 1 cup canned chickpeas, drained and rinsed)

3 tablespoons freshly squeezed lemon juice

¼ teaspoon sea salt

8 kalamata olives, pitted

1 cup frozen or canned artichoke hearts, chopped

2 tablespoons tahini

2 garlic cloves, peeled

Celery, carrots, and red bell pepper strips, for serving

If using frozen artichokes, pour boiling water over them to thaw; drain. Puree all of the dip ingredients until smooth. Serve with veggies.

Nutrition facts (per serving of dip): 32 calories; 1 g fat; 136 mg sodium; 4 g carbs; 1 g fiber; 1 g sugar; 1 g protein

Nutrition facts (per serving of dip with veggies): 88 calories; 2 g fat; 279 mg sodium; 16 g carbs; 5 g fiber; 7 g sugar; 3 g protein

ROASTED RED PEPPER HUMMUS

GF LC V DF

Makes 16 servings • Serving size: 2 tablespoons dip and 1 cup veggies

This hummus is a great way to get cancer- and inflammation-fighting cauliflower into your diet if you don't like the taste of it on its own. The roasted peppers take over the flavor and are an amazing source of vitamin C and antioxidants. If you want to switch things up, swap in sun-dried tomatoes for the red peppers.

1 cup canned chickpeas, drained and rinsed

½ cup **Cauliflower Base Blend** (page 84)

3 tablespoons chopped roasted red peppers

1 tablespoon freshly squeezed lemon juice

¼ teaspoon sea salt

2 tablespoons tahini

Carrots, celery, and red pepper strips, for serving

Puree all of the dip ingredients until smooth. Serve with veggies.

Nutrition facts (per serving of dip): 29 calories; 1 g fat; 132 mg sodium; 4 g carbs; 1 g fiber; 0 g sugar; 1 g protein

Nutrition facts (per serving of dip with veggies): 85 calories; 2 g fat; 275 mg sodium; 16 g carbs; 5 g fiber; 7 g sugar; 3 g protein

JUMPING BEAN DIP

Makes 8 servings • Serving size: 2 tablespoons dip and 1 tortilla, made into chips

GF
LC
V

This recipe is a slimmed-down version of refried beans. And it's lightened up even more by making your own fresh-baked tortilla chips. You'll never want to buy the bagged kind again.

1 cup **Black Bean–Blueberry–Baby Kale Base Blend** (page 100)

2 tablespoons plain low-fat Greek yogurt

1 tablespoon freshly squeezed lime juice

1 to 2 teaspoons chipotle chile in adobe sauce (or 2 tablespoons salsa)

Sea salt and freshly ground black pepper

8 6-inch sprouted corn tortillas, for serving

Extra-virgin olive oil

½ teaspoon chili powder (optional)

Preheat the oven to 400 degrees. Mix all of the dip ingredients in a medium bowl. Cut the tortillas into wedges or strips, mist or brush lightly with olive oil, and dust with a little chili powder, if using. Bake for about 10 minutes, until crisp. Serve the dip with the tortilla chips.

Nutrition facts (per serving of dip): 34 calories; 0 g fat; 23 mg sodium; 6 g carbs; 2 g fiber; 1 g sugar; 2 g protein

Nutrition facts (per serving of dip with tortilla chips): 94 calories; 1 g fat; 28 mg sodium; 19 g carbs; 4 g fiber; 1 g sugar; 4 g protein

LENTIL-CARROT CURRY DIP

(GF LC V DF)

Makes 8 servings • Serving size: 2 tablespoons dip and 6 lentil crackers

This dip was inspired by Indian dal, a lentil dish that's spiked with fragrant spices. Cook the lentils according to the package directions, and don't worry if they look more like a blend than lentils when you're done. They're much softer than black or green lentils, so that's how they're supposed to turn out.

½ cup cooked red or orange split lentils

½ cup **Carrot–Sweet Potato Base Blend** (page 86)

1 to 2 tablespoons curry powder

1 tablespoon extra-virgin olive oil

1 to 2 garlic cloves, peeled

Sea salt and freshly ground black pepper

48 lentil crackers, for serving

1 to 2 tablespoons chopped fresh cilantro

Puree the lentils, the blend, curry powder, olive oil, garlic, salt, and pepper until smooth. Stir in the cilantro. Serve with lentil crackers.

Nutrition facts (per serving of dip): 38 calories; 2 g fat; 7 mg sodium; 5 g carbs; 2 g fiber; 1 g sugar; 1 g protein

Nutrition facts (per serving of dip with lentil crackers): 109 calories; 5 g fat; 176 mg sodium; 14 g carbs; 3 g fiber; 1 g sugar; 4 g protein

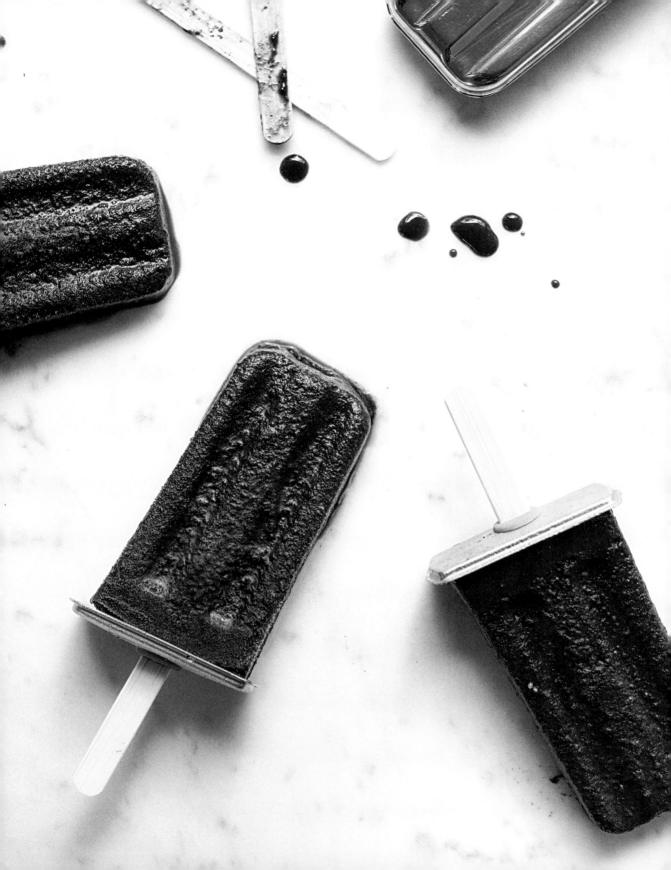

COFFEE-CHIA BREWSICLES

Makes 4 servings • Serving size: 1 popsicle

GF
V
DF

This is a great afternoon pick-me-up when you hit an energy low and need a little caffeine. Plus, the healthy fat and fiber in the avocado and the blend will sustain you until dinner. Tip: You can blend up extra servings of these pops and enjoy them as a refreshing, icy coffee drink, if you prefer.

1 teaspoon chia seeds

½ cup brewed coffee

1 cup **Blueberry–Baby Spinach Base Blend** (page 98)

¼ ripe avocado

1 to 2 tablespoons raw honey

Dash of ground cinnamon (optional)

Soak the chia seeds in the coffee for 5 minutes. Puree the coffee, chia seeds, and remaining ingredients until smooth. Pour into 4 popsicle molds (about ⅓ cup of coffee mixture each, depending on the size of your mold) and freeze.

Nutrition facts (per serving): 84 calories; 2 g fat; 28 mg sodium; 16 g carbs; 4 g fiber; 11 g sugar; 2 g protein

CREAMY WHITE BEAN "BUTTER" DIP

Makes 4 servings • Serving size: 2 tablespoons dip and 1 crostini

This is a great substitute for butter on bread—thus the "butter" in the recipe name—and it takes just a minute to make. So good!

1 cup **White Bean Base Blend** (page 83)

½ tablespoon extra-virgin olive oil

Juice of ½ lemon

1 garlic clove, minced

1 tablespoon minced fresh oregano and/or thyme

Sea salt and freshly ground black pepper

Small slices whole grain crostini, for serving

Put all of the ingredients for the dip into a medium bowl and whisk to combine. Serve the dip with the crostini.

Nutrition facts (per serving for dip): 96 calories; 3 g fat; 31 mg sodium; 14 g carbs; 4 g fiber; 0 g sugar; 5 g protein

Nutrition facts (per serving for dip with crostini): 145 calories; 4 g fat; 136 mg sodium; 23 g carbs; 6 g fiber; 1 g sugar; 8 g protein

Sip
Smoothies and Nourishing Drinks

Some of these drinks contain infusions of my blends; and others are more like heartier shakes, and can be eaten like a snack. When you have a blend on hand, it makes preparing a shake even faster and easier. This is where your blends become almost like those smoothie packs you see in the store, only better and fresher!

THE DRINK	THE BASE BLEND
Mixed Berry–Kale Shake	Mixed Berry–Baby Kale Base Blend (or Blueberry–Baby Spinach Base Blend)
Creamy Pumpkin Shake	Pumpkin Base Blend (or any Orange Base Blend)
Purple Detox Lemonade	Blueberry–Baby Spinach Base Blend (or Mixed Berry–Baby Kale Base Blend)
Winter Detox Hot Cocoa	Pumpkin Base Blend (or any Orange Base Blend)
Summer Zinger Detox	Raspberry-Beet Base Blend (or Raspberry Base Blend)

MIXED BERRY–KALE SHAKE

GF V

• *Makes 1 serving* •

½ cup frozen **Mixed Berry–Baby Kale Base Blend** (page 99)

1 teaspoon raw honey

1 tablespoon plain low-fat Greek yogurt

Blend all of the ingredients until smooth and serve.

Nutrition facts: 104 calories; 0 g fat; 26 mg sodium; 24 g carbs; 7 g fiber; 11 g sugar; 2 g protein

CREAMY PUMPKIN SHAKE

GF V

• *Makes 1 serving* •

½ cup **Pumpkin Base Blend** (page 88)

2 tablespoons plain low-fat Greek yogurt

½ tablespoon pure maple syrup

¼ teaspoon grated fresh ginger, or pinch of ground ginger

Pinch of sea salt

Pinch of ground cinnamon

Puree all of the ingredients and serve at room temperature.

Nutrition facts: 120 calories; 0 g fat; 240 mg sodium; 24 g carbs; 6 g fiber; 13 g sugar; 5 g protein

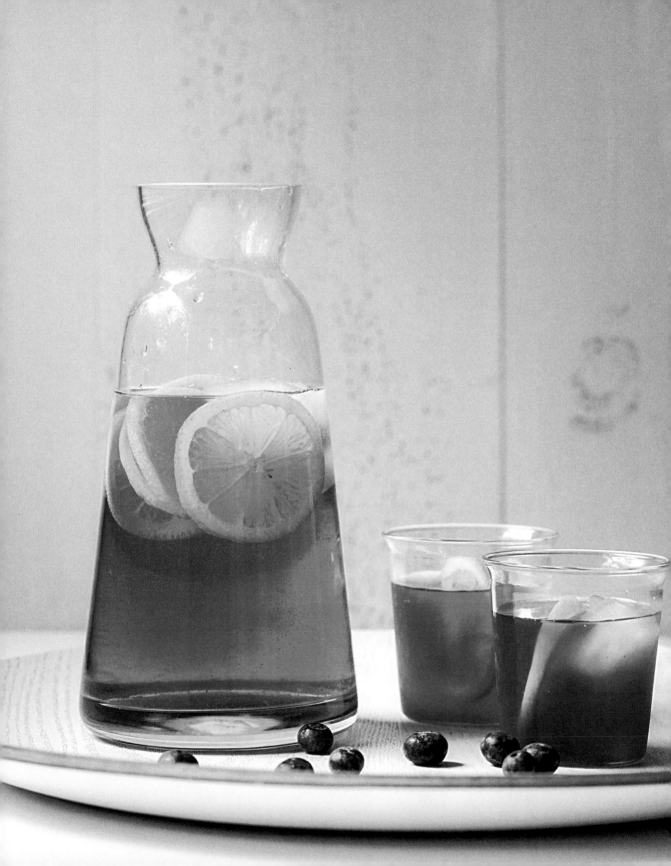

PURPLE DETOX LEMONADE

6F V DF

• Makes 1 serving •

Steep this lemonade as you would tea to infuse it with the goodness of the Blueberry–Baby Spinach Base Blend. Oh, and if you don't have this exact blend on hand, it works just as well to sub in 1 cup baby spinach and ½ cup frozen wild blueberries. I also love making ice cubes out of this lemonade; they add great flavor to water any time.

½ cup **Blueberry–Baby Spinach Base Blend** (page 98)

1 teaspoon raw honey

Juice of ½ lemon

1 cup boiling water

Stir all of the ingredients together and steep for 10 minutes, muddling occasionally. Pour through a fine-mesh strainer, discard the solids, and serve over ice.

Nutrition facts (per serving): 56 calories; 0 g fat; 37 mg sodium; 14 g carbs; 3 g fiber; 8 g sugar; 1 g protein

GF
V
DF

WINTER DETOX HOT COCOA

• Makes 1 serving •

I love to have this as an afternoon snack. It feels so comforting and warming, but it also has the cleansing powers of cinnamon, ginger, and cocoa. And the pumpkin makes it rich and creamy. Way better for you than those trendy pumpkin spice lattes that don't even use real pumpkin, and weigh in at 300 calories a serving.

¼ teaspoon ground cinnamon

¼ teaspoon freshly grated
  peeled ginger

½ tablespoon unsweetened
  cocoa powder

¼ cup **Pumpkin Base Blend**
  (page 88)

1 to 2 teaspoons raw honey

½ cup unsweetened coconut
  or almond milk

¼ cup water

¼ teaspoon pure vanilla
  extract

Warm all of the ingredients in a small pot over medium heat; bring to a simmer and serve.

Nutrition facts (per serving): 105 calories; 3 g fat; 14 mg sodium; 20 g carbs; 6 g fiber; 13 g sugar; 3 g protein

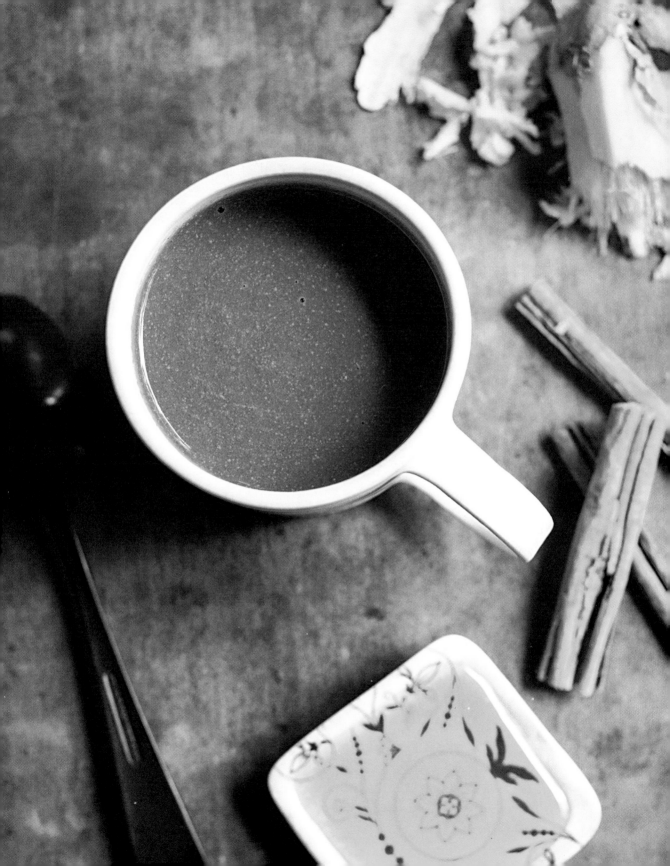

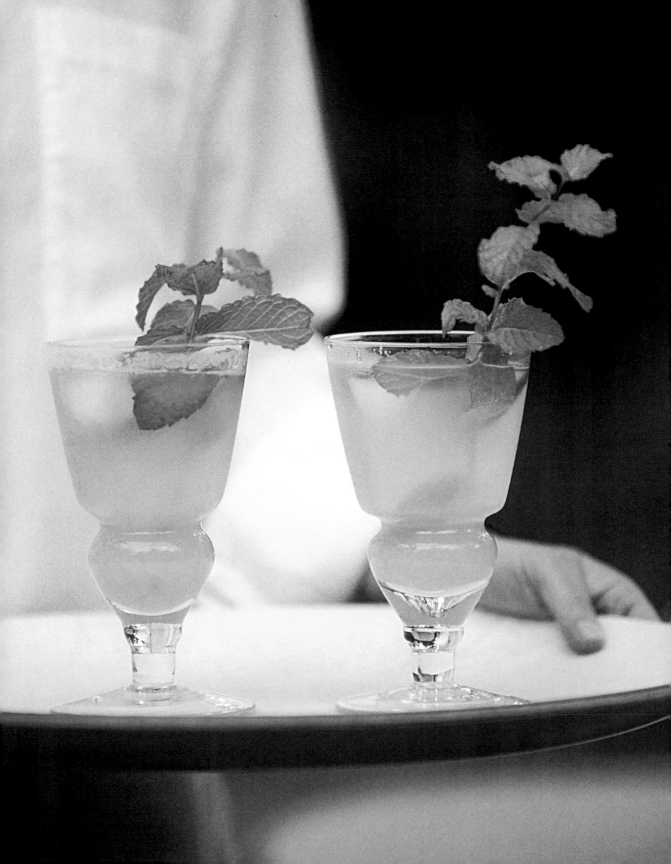

CUCUMBER-LIME DETOX SODA

• Makes 1 serving •

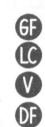

Cucumber and lime are a classic cleansing flavor combo. It's like a spa in a glass! I can't get enough of this drink. Want to make it even more special? It's super-refreshing served in an ice-cold martini glass on a hot summer day.

1 medium cucumber, peeled
   and seeded

Juice of ½ lime

1 cup sparkling mineral water

Sprig of fresh mint

Puree the cucumber and pour through a fine-mesh strainer, discarding the solids. Add the remaining ingredients and serve over ice.

Nutrition facts (per serving): 15 calories; 0 g fat; 1 mg sodium; 4 g carbs; 1 g fiber; 1 g sugar; 0 g protein

SUMMER ZINGER DETOX

• *Makes 2 servings* •

This refreshing drink is great any time, but it's particularly good after a tough workout. Beets are touted to improve blood and oxygen flow to your muscles to help you recover; and some athletes believe beets also boosts their performance. No wonder they're a go-to among pros.

½ cup **Raspberry-Beet Base Blend** (page 94)

Zest and juice of 1 lemon

1-inch piece of fresh ginger, peeled and roughly chopped

1 to 2 teaspoons pure maple syrup

2 cups boiling water

Place the first 4 ingredients in a heatproof bowl. Pour the boiling water over the mixture and steep for 5 minutes, muddling occasionally. Pour through a fine-mesh strainer, discarding the solids, and serve over ice.

Nutrition facts (per serving): 41 calories; 0 g fat; 12 mg sodium; 14 g carbs; 3 g fiber; 9 g sugar; 1 g protein

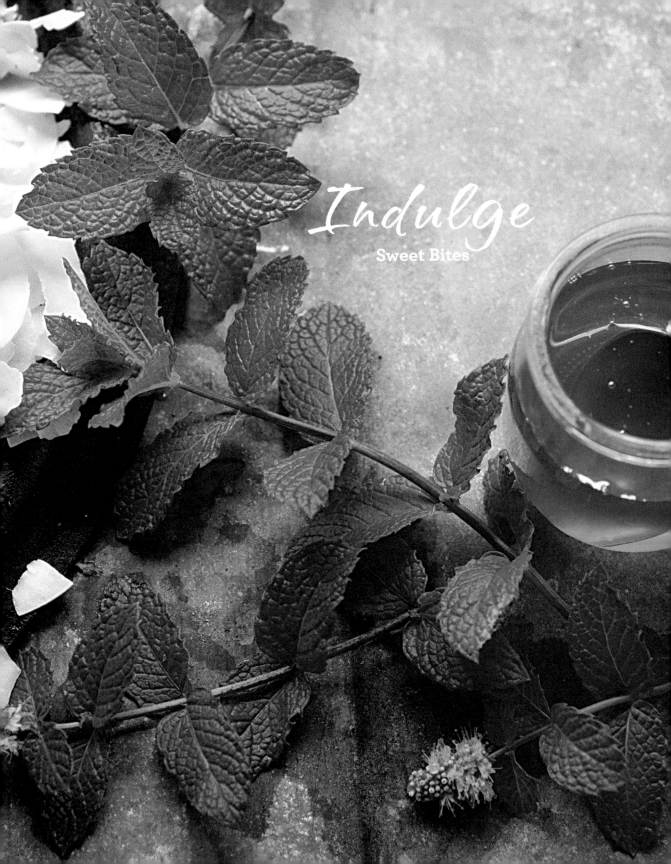

Indulge

Sweet Bites

So many diets forbid sweets and desserts, period—and I totally get why. Usually, they're loaded with butter, refined sugar, cream, and an obscene number of calories. But with my blends, you can actually have your cake—and whoopie pies and brownies—and eat it, too. That's because my blends stand in for much of the fat and sweetener in a recipe, slashing calories while simultaneously making something that should be a sugar bomb into something that's truly nutritious. Dessert just got the green light again!

The chart below allows you to choose a recipe based on a blend you have on hand—and gives you alternative options to the blend I call for in the recipe, to make the recipes even more versatile.

THE DISH	THE BASE BLEND
Mixed Berry Sorbet Blend	Mixed Berry–Baby Kale Base Blend
Mango Lassi Sorbet	Butternut Squash–Apple Base Blend
Frosted Banana Cupcake Bites	Carrot–Sweet Potato Base Blend (or any Orange Base Blend)
Gluten-Free Banana Cupcake Bites	Butternut Squash–Apple Base Blend (or any Orange Base Blend)
45-Calorie Pumpkin Whoopie Pies	Pumpkin Base Blend (or any Orange Base Blend)
Un-Devilish Devil Dogs	Beet Base Blend (or Raspberry-Beet Base Blend)
5-a-Day Brownies	Mixed Berry–Baby Kale Base Blend or Carrot–Sweet Potato Base Blend (or any Purple and Orange Base Blend)
Cinnamon-Oat Truffle Treats	White Bean Base Blend
Coconut-Almond Truffle Treats	White Bean Base Blend
Cocoa-Cayenne Truffle Treats	White Bean Base Blend
Skinny Chocolate Cake	Black Bean–Blueberry–Baby Kale Base Blend (or any Purple Base Blend)
Puree Brûlée	Carrot–Sweet Potato Base Blend (or Pumpkin Base Blend)
Frozen Fudge Pops	Raspberry Base Blend

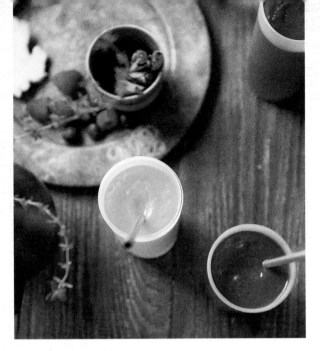

1-MINUTE DESSERT

Yes, my blends even make yummy desserts! Add a couple extra ingredients and you can transform a Base Blend into an indulgent after-dinner treat in no time—one that also happens to be incredibly good for you.

MIXED BERRY SORBET BLEND

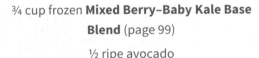

Makes 4 servings • Serving size: $^{1}/_{2}$ cup

¾ cup frozen **Mixed Berry–Baby Kale Base Blend** (page 99)

½ ripe avocado

2 teaspoons raw honey

Cold filtered water

Thaw the blend slightly, then put it with the avocado and the honey into a high-powered blender and puree until smooth, adding a little water as necessary to make a thick sorbet. Serve in parfait glasses. If you want a firmer consistency, freeze for 30 minutes.

Nutrition facts (per serving): 67 calories; 3 g fat; 12 mg sodium; 11 g carbs; 4 g fiber; 6 g sugar; 1 g protein

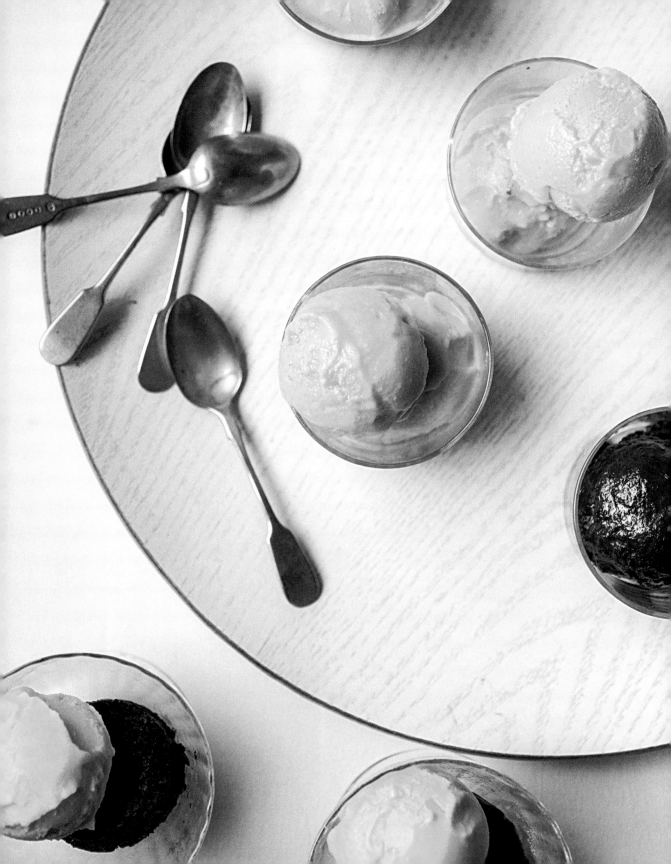

MANGO LASSI SORBET

Makes 4 servings • Serving size: ¹/₂ cup

I gave this traditional Indian drink a twist by turning it into an exotic-tasting sorbet. If you don't have Butternut Squash–Apple Base Blend in your fridge or freezer, you can use ¼ cup frozen squash and one quarter of a fresh, peeled and cored apple.

⅓ cup **Butternut Squash–Apple Base Blend** (page 87)

1 ½ cups diced frozen mango

¼ cup plain low-fat Greek yogurt

2 to 3 tablespoons low-fat milk or unsweetened coconut milk

Pinch of ground cardamom, or more to taste

2 teaspoons raw honey

Cold filtered water

Puree all of the ingredients until smooth, adding a little water as necessary to make a thick sorbet. Serve in parfait glasses. If you want a firmer consistency, freeze for 30 minutes.

Nutrition facts (per serving): 75 calories; 0 g fat; 9 mg sodium; 18 g carbs; 2 g fiber; 15 g sugar; 2 g protein

MINT CHOCOLATE
CHIP GELATO

Makes 4 servings • Serving size: 1/2 cup

Who needs nasty—and unhealthy—food coloring when you can get a beautiful green color naturally? The mint hue in this gelato comes from avocado and spinach—which you'll never taste—and the real mint adds a coolness and pop of flavor that the faux stuff could never deliver.

2 frozen bananas, chopped (about 2 cups)

¼ ripe avocado

¼ cup baby spinach

¼ cup unsweetened almond or coconut milk (or low-fat milk)

A few sprigs of fresh mint

1 to 2 teaspoons raw honey

1 to 2 tablespoons cocoa nibs

Puree the first 6 ingredients until smooth. (Use a smaller amount of milk if you want a thicker soft-serve consistency.) Stir in the cocoa nibs. If you want a firmer gelato, freeze the mixture for at least 1 hour before scooping.

Nutrition facts (per serving): 104 calories; 4 g fat; 22 mg sodium; 20 g carbs; 3 g fiber; 12 g sugar; 1 g protein

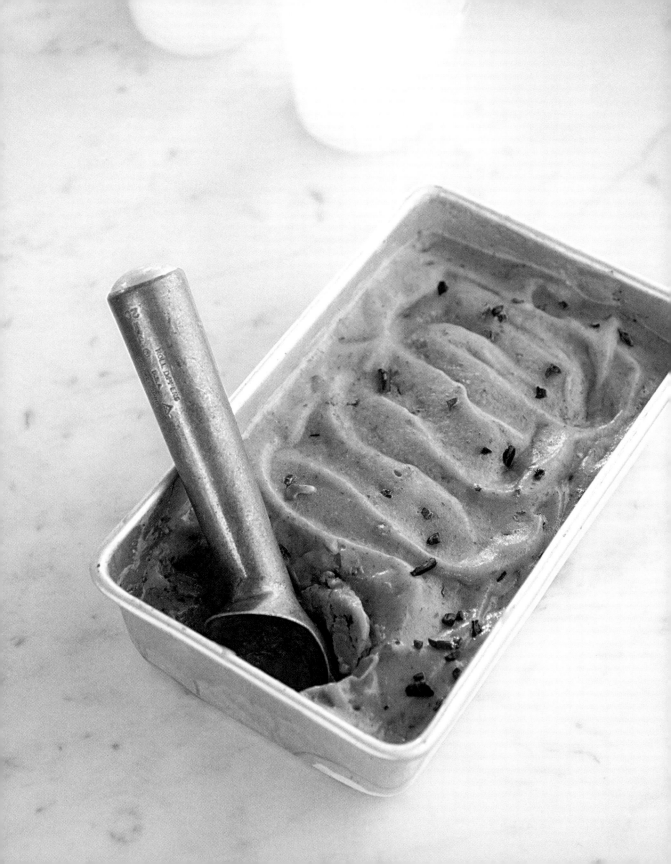

PB AND BANANA GELATO

Makes 4 servings • Serving size: ¹/₂ cup

Full disclosure: This dessert is one of the few in this book that doesn't include a Base Blend; but it's so delicious I couldn't not include it. It has no eggs or heavy cream and provides more nutrition than pretty much any gelato or ice cream ever. If you don't have frozen bananas on hand, you can chop up fresh bananas and throw them into the freezer for an hour before making the gelato.

2 frozen bananas, chopped
(about 2 cups)

¼ cup plain low-fat Greek
yogurt

1 tablespoon natural creamy
peanut butter (or Sneaky
Chef No-Nut Butter)

1 tablespoon raw honey

Puree all of the ingredients until smooth. If you want a firmer gelato, freeze the mixture for at least 1 hour before scooping.

Nutrition facts (per serving): 100 calories; 2 g fat; 24 mg sodium; 19 g carbs; 2 g fiber; 12 g sugar; 3 g protein

FROSTED BANANA CUPCAKE BITES

Makes about 15 servings • Serving size: 2 cupcake bites

Who needs buttercream? The frosting in this recipe is a variation of my DIY Cream Cheese—and it's delicious. Strain the Greek yogurt for the frosting in the fridge while you get everything else ready and it will be good to go by the time the cupcakes are done. If you're a big chocolate lover like me, you can swap in the frosting from the Gluten-Free Banana Cupcake Bites on page 236 if you like. (Refrigerate any extra cupcakes, because the frosting is perishable.)

For the frosting

¼ cup plain low-fat Greek yogurt

½ ripe banana, mashed

1 tablespoon raw honey

For the cupcakes

Nonstick cooking spray

1 cup plus 1 tablespoon whole grain pastry flour

¼ teaspoon ground cinnamon

¼ teaspoon sea salt

1 teaspoon baking powder

¼ cup canola or light olive oil

¼ cup pure maple syrup

1 large egg

¼ cup low-fat milk

½ cup **Carrot–Sweet Potato Base Blend** (page 86)

1 banana, mashed

1 teaspoon pure vanilla extract

(Recipe continued on next page)

Make the frosting: Put the yogurt in a strainer lined with paper towels and allow to strain over a bowl for 30 minutes to thicken. In a small bowl, whisk the strained yogurt with the banana and honey.

Meanwhile, make the cupcakes: Preheat the oven to 350 degrees. Mist a mini donut or mini muffin tin with cooking spray. In a large bowl, whisk together the flour, cinnamon, salt, and baking powder. In another bowl, combine the oil, maple syrup, egg, milk, the blend, banana, and vanilla. Stir the dry mixture into the wet ingredients until just combined. Spoon the batter into the baking tin, filling each individual well about three-quarters full. Bake for 16 minutes, until a toothpick inserted into the center of a cupcake comes out clean; set aside to cool completely. Spread 1 teaspoon of the frosting over each cupcake.

Nutrition facts (per serving): 103 calories; 4 g fat; 82 mg sodium; 15 g carbs; 1 g fiber; 6 g sugar; 2 g protein

GLUTEN-FREE BANANA CUPCAKE BITES

Makes about 15 servings • Serving size: 2 cupcakes

These cupcakes make a great bite-size treat—and we all know two is always better than one, even if they're mini. If you don't have a mini cupcake tin to make these in, it's worth the small investment. I know it seems like a super-specialized item that you'll only use once, but I honestly bust mine out for everything from mini meatballs to frittatas. They cook faster and are totally adorable. Let the cupcakes cool completely before frosting them; this will also give you time to let the yogurt in the frosting strain. (Refrigerate any extra cupcakes, because the frosting is perishable.)

For the frosting

½ cup plain low-fat Greek yogurt

2 tablespoons raw honey

2 teaspoons unsweetened cocoa powder

¼ cup cocoa nibs (optional)

For the cupcakes

Nonstick cooking spray

1 cup plus 1 tablespoon gluten-free flour

¼ teaspoon ground cinnamon

¼ teaspoon sea salt

1 teaspoon baking powder

¼ cup canola oil

1 large egg

1 teaspoon pure vanilla extract

2 tablespoons pure maple syrup

½ cup **Butternut Squash–Apple Base Blend** (page 87)

1 banana, mashed

Make the frosting: Place the yogurt in a strainer lined with paper towels and allow to strain over a bowl for 30 minutes to thicken. In a small bowl, whisk the strained yogurt with the honey and cocoa.

Meanwhile, make the cupcakes: Preheat oven to 350 degrees. Mist a mini donut or mini muffin tin with cooking spray. In a large bowl, whisk together the flour, cinnamon, salt, and baking powder. In another bowl, combine the oil, egg, vanilla, maple syrup, the blend, and the banana. Stir the dry mixture into the wet ingredients until just combined. Spoon the batter into the baking tin, filling each individual well about three-quarters full. Bake for 16 minutes, until a toothpick inserted into the center of a cupcake comes out clean; set aside to cool completely. Spread 1 teaspoon of the frosting over each cupcake and sprinkle with 3 or 4 cocoa nibs, if using.

Nutrition facts (per serving): 106 calories; 6 g fat; 97 mg sodium; 14 g carbs; 2 g fiber; 4 g sugar; 2 g protein

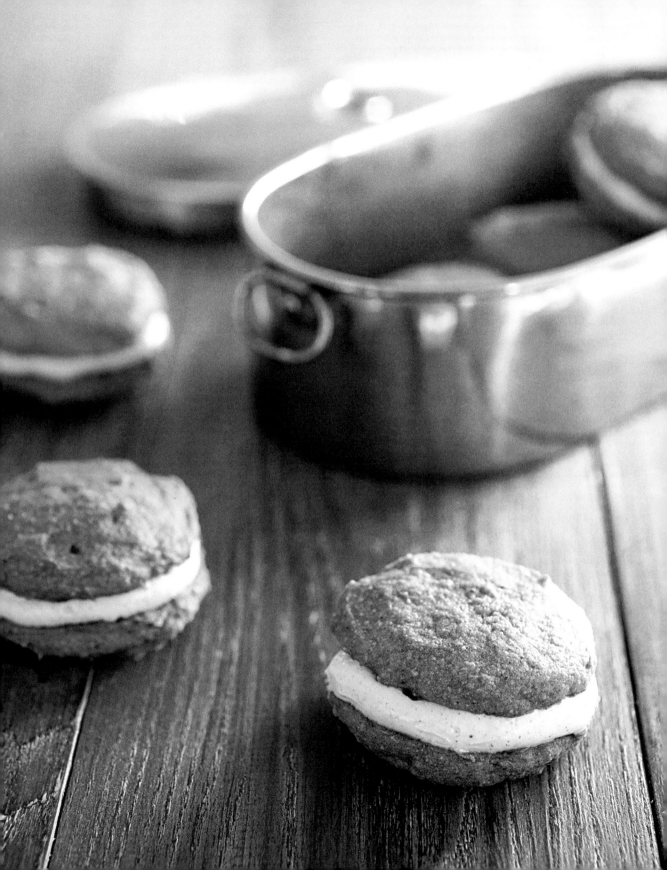

45-CALORIE PUMPKIN WHOOPIE PIES

Makes 24 servings • Serving size: 1 whoopie pie

Yep, you read that right: Each of these incredibly moist, evil-looking whoopie pies is only 45 calories. And they're truly healthy, too. If you don't have whole grain pastry flour, you can use white whole wheat flour or half whole wheat flour and half all-purpose flour—but don't use all whole wheat flour or they won't be as light and fluffy.

For the filling

1 ½ cups plain low-fat Greek yogurt

2 tablespoons pure maple syrup

½ teaspoon pumpkin pie spice or ground cinnamon

1 teaspoon pure vanilla extract

For the pies

2 tablespoons canola or light olive oil

1 large egg

½ teaspoon pure vanilla extract

¾ cup **Pumpkin Base Blend** (page 88)

⅓ cup pure maple syrup

¾ teaspoon pumpkin pie spice

½ teaspoon sea salt

½ teaspoon baking soda

¾ cup, plus 2 tablespoons whole grain pastry flour

1 teaspoon baking powder

Make the filling: Put the yogurt in a strainer lined with paper towels and allow to strain over a bowl for 30 minutes to thicken. In a small bowl, whisk the strained yogurt with the maple syrup, pumpkin pie spice, and vanilla.

Meanwhile, make the pies: Preheat the oven to 350 degrees. Line two baking sheets with parchment paper. In a medium bowl, add the oil, egg, vanilla, the blend, and the maple syrup. In another bowl, combine the pumpkin pie spice, salt, baking soda, flour, and baking powder. Stir the dry mixture into the wet ingredients until just combined. Drop 1 scant teaspoon of the batter onto the baking sheets, leaving a few inches between them (try to make them rounded). Bake for about 12 minutes, or until the pies are springy when you press the top; set aside to cool completely. Spread 1 tablespoon of the filling on one pie and top with another one to make a sandwich.

Nutrition facts (per serving): 45 calories; 2 g fat; 102 mg sodium; 6 g carbs; 1 g fiber; 2 g sugar; 2 g protein

UN-DEVILISH DEVIL DOGS

Makes 24 servings • Serving size: 1 sandwich

I grew up with Devil Dogs; truth be told, they were almost a main food group for me. (If only I'd known then how devilish they really were!) The shape of these is a little different, but wow does the taste take me back. Only with my recipe, you're getting tons of antioxidants from the beets and cherries. They also have zero preservatives, unlike their million-year-shelf-life counterpart has. Note: Whole grain pastry flour is whole wheat flour that's been ground into an ultra-fine powder, which produces a fluffier treat—and is an excellent source of fiber. If you're stuck, use a half-and-half mix of whole wheat flour and all-purpose.

For the Filling

1 ½ cups plain low-fat Greek yogurt

2 tablespoons pure maple syrup

1 teaspoon pure vanilla extract

For the Cakes

2 tablespoons canola or light olive oil

1 large egg

1 teaspoon pure vanilla extract

¼ cup **Beet Base Blend** (page 96) (or
  ¾ cup **Raspberry-Beet Base Blend**
  [page 99], and omit the cherries)

¾ cup frozen pitted sweet cherries,
  pureed with a little water

⅓ cup pure maple syrup

½ teaspoon sea salt

½ teaspoon baking soda

1 cup whole grain pastry flour

2 tablespoons unsweetened cocoa
  powder

¼ teaspoon ground coffee or espresso

1 teaspoon baking powder

Make the filling first: Place the yogurt in a strainer lined with paper towels and allow to strain over a bowl for 30 minutes to thicken. In a small bowl, whisk the strained yogurt with the maple syrup and vanilla.

Meanwhile, make the cakes: Preheat the oven to 350 degrees. Line 2 baking sheets with parchment paper. In a medium bowl, add the oil, egg, vanilla, the blend, the cherry puree, and the maple syrup. In another bowl, combine the salt, baking soda, flour, cocoa, coffee, and baking powder. Stir the dry mixture into the wet ingredients until just combined. Drop scant teaspoons of the batter onto the baking sheets, leaving a few inches between them (try to make them rounded). Bake for about 12 minutes, or until the cakes are springy when you press the top; set aside to cool completely. Spread 1 tablespoon of the filling on one cake and top with another one to make a sandwich.

Nutrition facts (per serving): 60 calories; 2 g fat; 104 mg sodium; 10 g carbs; 1 g fiber; 5 g sugar; 2 g protein

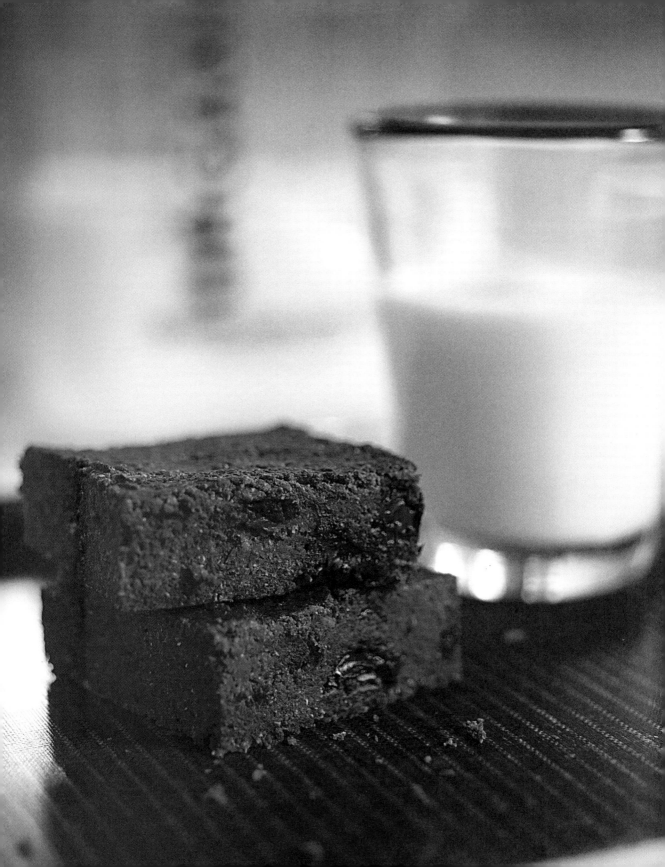

5-A-DAY BROWNIES

Makes 16 servings • Serving size: 1 brownie

These brownies feature five different fruits and veggies: blueberries, raspberries, kale, carrots, and sweet potato. And they are made with whole grains. But your taste buds will only register the rich, fudgy brownie part. I usually don't call for two different blends in a recipe, but they allow you to replace nearly all of the oil and sugar—making this a brownie that's incredibly good for you.

1 large egg

6 tablespoons canola or light olive oil

⅓ cup raw honey

1 teaspoon pure vanilla extract

¼ teaspoon sea salt

¼ teaspoon baking soda

¼ cup unsweetened cocoa powder

½ cup **Mixed Berry–Baby Kale Base Blend** (page 99)

⅓ cup **Carrot–Sweet Potato Base Blend** (page 86)

⅓ cup dark chocolate chips

1 cup whole grain pastry flour

Nonstick cooking spray

Preheat the oven to 350 degrees. In a large bowl, whisk together the first 9 ingredients. Stir in the chocolate chips and flour. Mist an 8 x 8-inch metal or glass baking dish with the cooking spray and spread the batter evenly in the dish. (If using a glass dish, lower the oven temperature by 25 degrees.) Bake for 33 to 35 minutes, until a toothpick inserted into the center comes out clean and the brownies begin to pull away from the sides of the pan.

Nutrition facts (per serving): 131 calories; 7 g fat; 79 mg sodium; 17 g carbs; 2 g fiber; 9 g sugar; 2 g protein

CINNAMON-OAT TRUFFLE TREATS

Makes 8 servings • Serving size: 2 truffles

These treats, which were in the Reboot, reappear here because they are—by far—the favorite thing in this book among anyone who has ever tried them. People are obsessed with these, myself included. I have them in my freezer at all times. Freezing them makes the truffle treats even better, and forces you to slow down and savor them longer—so they seem even more satisfying.

6 tablespoons **White Bean Base Blend** (page 83)

½ cup almond butter (or Sneaky Chef No-Nut Butter)

1 tablespoon 100% fruit, no-sugar-added jam

2 tablespoons ground flaxseed meal

½ cup finely ground rolled oats, divided (or gluten-free oats)

½ teaspoon ground cinnamon

Pinch of sea salt

On a plate, mix the blend, almond butter, jam, flaxseed, and 2 tablespoons of the oats until well combined. On another plate, mix the remaining oats with the cinnamon and salt. Use a melon baller or measuring spoon to make tablespoon-size balls of the blend mixture. Roll the truffles in the cinnamon-oat mixture. Serve right away, or place the truffles in a container and freeze for at least 30 minutes before serving.

Nutrition facts (per serving): 144 calories; 11 g fat; 6 mg sodium; 11 g carbs; 2 g fiber; 1 g sugar; 4 g protein

* *(if using gluten-free oats)*

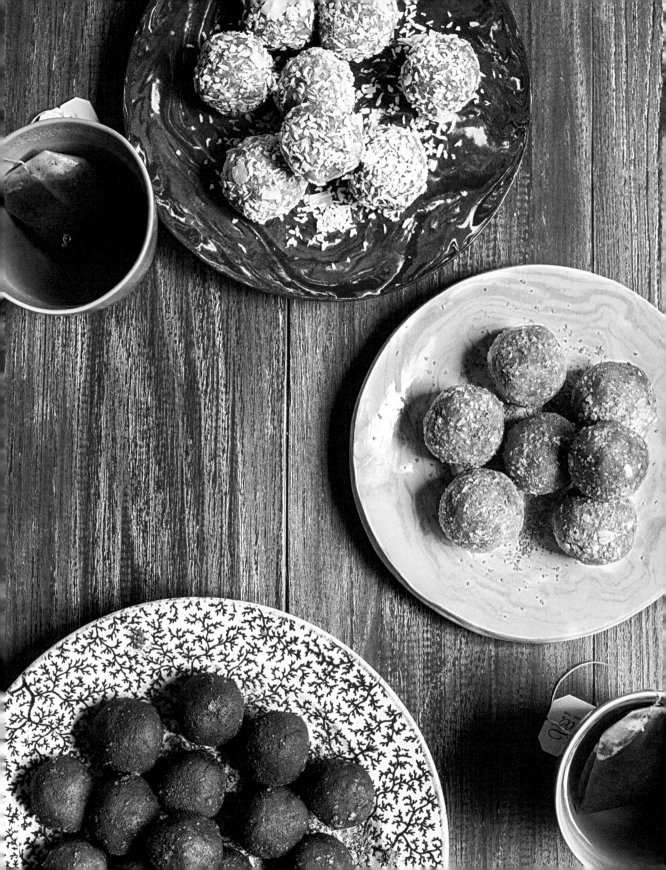

COCONUT-ALMOND TRUFFLE TREATS

Makes 8 servings • Serving size: 2 truffles

My original truffle treats were so popular that I developed other variations of them, to keep things interesting. I like to freeze them—otherwise, they're so yummy I'd be tempted to gobble them all in two seconds.

6 tablespoons **White Bean Base Blend** (page 83)

½ cup almond butter (or Sneaky Chef No-Nut Butter)

¼ cup finely ground rolled oats, divided (or gluten-free oats)

1 tablespoon raw honey

¼ cup unsweetened coconut flakes

On a plate, mix the first 4 ingredients until well combined. Place the coconut on another plate. Use a melon baller or measuring spoon to make tablespoon-size balls of the blend mixture. Roll the truffles in the coconut, pressing lightly to help them stick. Serve right away, or place the truffles in a container and freeze for at least 30 minutes before serving.

Nutrition facts (per serving): 150 calories; 12 g fat; 7 mg sodium; 10 g carbs; 1 g fiber; 3 g sugar; 4 g protein

* *(if using gluten-free oats)*

COCOA-CAYENNE TRUFFLE TREATS

Makes 8 servings • Serving size: 2 truffles

Cayenne may seem like a surprising ingredient, but it's such a brilliant flavor combo with cocoa. Bonus: The compound that gives cayenne pepper its kick—called capsaicin—has been shown to increase metabolism and boost fat burning.

6 tablespoons **White Bean Base Blend** (page 83)

½ cup almond butter (or Sneaky Chef No-Nut Butter)

¾ cup finely ground rolled oats, divided (or gluten-free oats)

1 tablespoon raw honey

1 teaspoon unsweetened cocoa powder, divided

⅛ teaspoon cayenne pepper

On a plate, mix the blend, almond butter, 3 tablespoons of the oats, the honey, ½ teaspoon of the cocoa, and a pinch of the cayenne until well combined. On another plate, mix the remaining oats, cocoa, and remaining cayenne. Use a melon baller or measuring spoon to make tablespoon-size balls of the blend mixture. Roll the truffles in the cocoa-oat mixture. Serve right away, or place the truffles in a container and freeze for at least 30 minutes before serving.

Nutrition facts (per serving): 150 calories; 10 g fat; 7 mg sodium; 13 g carbs; 2 g fiber; 2 g sugar; 4 g protein

* *(if using gluten-free oats)*

SKINNY CHOCOLATE CAKE

Makes 12 servings • Serving size: 1 slice

This ooey-gooey, dense chocolate cake is also gluten free. And the Black Bean–Blueberry–Baby Kale Base Blend totally disappears in all that deliciousness, yet somehow adds an incredible depth of flavor. Note: If you've never baked with almond meal before, you can find it in the baking or nut aisle of almost every grocery store these days.

Nonstick cooking spray

3 ounces good dark chocolate

2 large eggs

¼ teaspoon sea salt

½ teaspoon almond extract

1 tablespoon coconut oil

½ cup **Black Bean–Blueberry–Baby Kale Base Blend** (page 100)

1 tablespoon unsweetened cocoa powder

¼ cup raw honey

½ cup plus 2 tablespoons almond meal *

Preheat the oven to 325 degrees. Mist a 9-inch round cake pan with cooking spray and set aside. Place a small heatproof bowl over a pot of simmering water to make a double boiler and add the chocolate, stirring often, until it melts; remove from the heat and allow to cool slightly. In a medium bowl, mix the remaining ingredients until well combined, then stir in the melted chocolate. Transfer to the prepared pan and bake for 30 to 32 minutes, until a toothpick inserted into the center comes out clean.

* If you can't find almond meal at the store, it's easy to make. Soak raw almonds (with the skins still on) overnight, drain, dry, then pulse them in a food processor until they form a meal-like consistency.

Nutrition facts (per serving): 122 calories; 7 g fat; 62 mg sodium; 13 g carbs; 2 g fiber; 10 g sugar; 3 g protein

PUREE BRÛLÉE

Makes 2 servings • Serving size: 1 brûlée

Regular crème brûlée is basically a dish of cream with a crust of sugar on top of it—neither of which exactly screams "diet" or "healthy." I found a way to get a similar look and creamy, rich taste, only so much lighter and easier to make. Each one has just 42 calories: It's like magic!

½ cup **Carrot–Sweet Potato Base Blend** (page 86)

½ teaspoon light olive oil

½ teaspoon pure vanilla extract

Pinch of sea salt

1 packet stevia (½ teaspoon)

Nonstick cooking spray

1 large egg white

⅛ teaspoon cream of tartar

Preheat the broiler. Whisk together the blend, oil, vanilla, salt, and half of the stevia packet (¼ teaspoon) in a medium bowl. Mist 2 ramekins with cooking spray and pour in the mixture. In another bowl, vigorously whisk the egg white, cream of tartar, and remaining stevia until foamy, then pour on top of the puree mixture. Broil for 4 to 5 minutes, until the top is browned and hardened. Serve warm or cooled.

Nutrition facts (per serving): 42 calories; 1 g fat; 52 mg sodium; 6 g carbs; 1 g fiber; 2 g sugar; 2 g protein

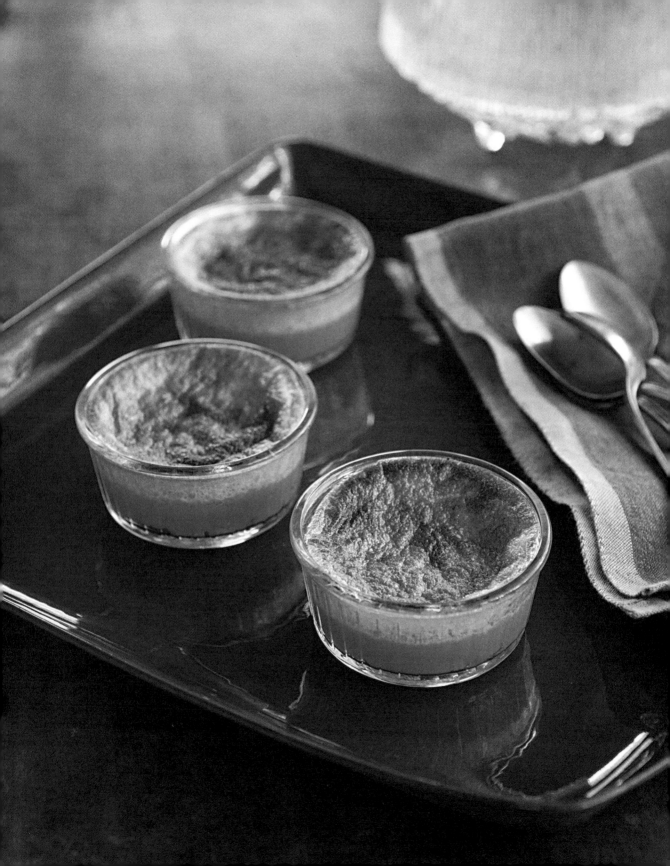

FROZEN FUDGE POPS

Makes 8 servings • Serving size: 1 fudgsicle

Anything you eat off a stick is instantly more fun; and this childhood throw-back is so yummy and chocolaty that it's hard to imagine it's actually packed with antioxidants, omegas, and fiber. I have to fight my kids for these!

2 teaspoons chia seeds

1½ cups unsweetened almond milk

½ ripe avocado

1 banana

1 tablespoon raw honey

1½ tablespoons unsweetened cocoa powder

Dash of ground cinnamon

½ cup **Raspberry Base Blend** (page 95)

Soak the chia seeds in the almond milk for 10 minutes while you prep the other ingredients. Put all the ingredients into a high-powered blender and puree until smooth. Freeze in 8 popsicle molds (about ⅓ cup of the mixture per popsicle, depending on the size of your mold) for at least 2 hours before serving.

Nutrition facts (per serving): 59 calories; 3 g fat; 34 mg sodium; 10 g carbs; 3 g fiber; 6 g sugar; 1 g protein

Join The Sneaky Blends Nation

By now you're a pro at incorporating Sneaky Blends into your life. I hope you've become as hooked on using them as I am—and that they will remain a permanent staple in your kitchen, because they offer so many amazing benefits. They're helping you save around 2,500 calories a week, you're able to eat all of your favorite foods, you're fulfilling your fiber requirements and easily getting all of your servings of fruits and veggies. You're also able to effortlessly maintain your weight or maybe even drop those extra pounds. There's an incredible amount of evidence that people who eat more fruits and veggies live longer and better—and by now you are Exhibit A of that fact. The blends you're using are a way to help prevent illness, while also bringing pure pleasure to your table.

Keep playing with new ways of adding blends to every dish you make, and become a part of the Sneaky Blends community by sharing your story, tips, and ideas with other blend devotees on my Facebook page: facebook.com/TheSneakyChef. Healthy eating plans are always easier to stick to when you have like-minded people supporting you and cheering you on. Tag your posts with #sneakyblends, #blends, or #blendscleanse. Check out my website, TheSneakyChef.com/SneakyBlends for new recipes, healthy products, and loads of blending inspiration.

Here's to health, wellness, and a lifetime of blending for all.

Join Our Online Community! Get Support and Connect With Other Blend Devotees On Facebook: facebook.com/TheSneakyChef.Missy.

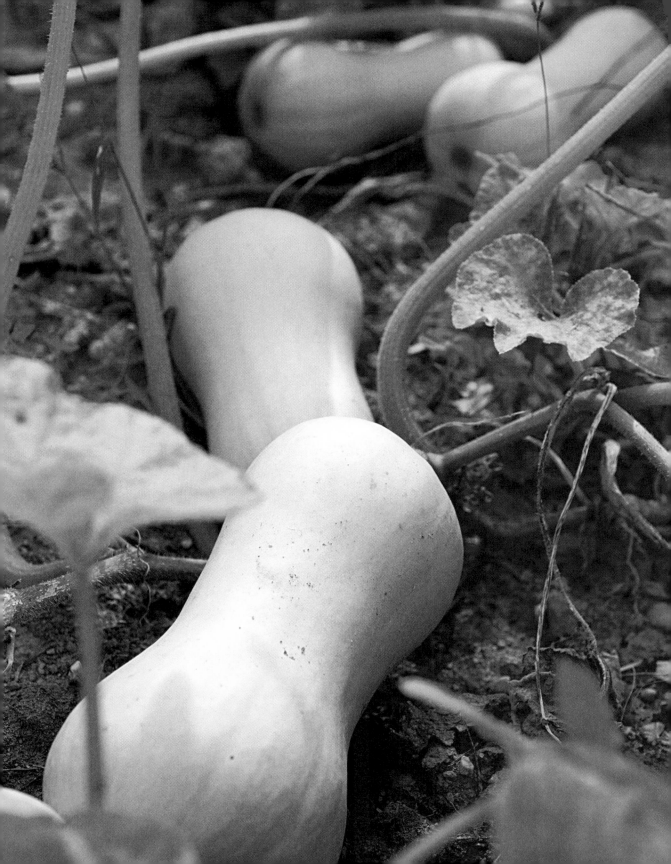

Acknowledgments

Writing this acknowledgments page makes sneaking veggies into my favorite foods seem easy! Words can't fully express how grateful I am for the support team of incredible talent around me—and the love and encouragement of my inner circle of family and friends. I am so thankful to each and every one of you!

Huge thanks to my always supportive and visionary literary agent Joelle Delbourgo, for believing in me from the birth of The Sneaky Chef and throughout this wonderful journey. You are a true friend and partner.

To my exceptional publishing team at North Star Way: My publisher, Michele Martin, for her incredible acumen and belief in me; my talented editors, Kathy Huck, Diana Ventimiglia, and Sophia Muthuraj; managing editor Irene Kheradi; copyediting director Navorn Johnson; copyeditor Janet McDonald; cover designer Laywan Kwan; designer Jaime Putorti; marketing associate Hilary Mau; and the entire talented team at Simon & Schuster, who understood the vision of this book from the start and stayed true to its message.

To my writing partner, Shaun Dreisbach, for your expertise and guidance. I could not have done this book without you.

Right by my side throughout this process has also been a group of people who constantly inspired and cheered me on: My mother, who taught me that food is love—and our best medicine. Thank you for working side by side with me, testing every recipe countless times. To my sister, Karen, whose friendship and support mean so much to me. And to my brother and spiritual twin, Larry, and Brigitte Chase, who have been my partners in crime since the very first notion of Sneaky Chef.

Special thanks to my dad, who instilled in me the work ethic and tenacity to follow my dreams; and to my stepmother, Ulla, an amazing cook who makes everything taste great and generously shares her secrets with me.

The mouthwatering food photos in this book are the excellent work and creative genius of food photographer Jennifer May, and Jennifer's team—food stylist Kendra McKnight, prop stylist Raina Kattelson, and assistant Sarah Honey Daniels. Thank you as well to the Hearty Roots Community Farm in Germantown, NY, for letting us raid your fields for farm-fresh vegetables—several times—over our weeklong shoot.

I am so grateful for the love and support of dear friends Risa and Steve Goldberg, Denise Gotsdiner and Andy Clibanoff, Sharon Hammer and Jeff Tamarin, Petra Kaufman and Tassos Koumbourlis, Laura Klein and Frank Rimler, Carolyn Kremins and Rob Rosenthal, Abby and Bruce Mendelsohn, Lisa Jacobson and Richard Lubarsky, and Tina Rosengarten.

Thank you to my kids and their besties—who were my tireless team of taste testers, and whose excitement and enthusiasm inspired my creativity in the kitchen.

I will always be grateful to my partners who helped me bring Sneaky Chef Foods into stores: Hellen Spanjer; Michael Carley; Matthew Glass; Paul Greenberg; and Jordan Sulkin. And to Steven Gelerman, Jeff Canner, Julie Kligman, and Melissa Drahzal at Action Brand Management and to Addis design: Steven Addis; Joanne Hom and Jonathan Fisher; and the entire product team for bringing Sneaky Chef Foods to store shelves and kitchens nationwide.

Thank you to my wonderful test kitchen manager, Jean Bukhan, who keeps me calm and organized—and to my personal business manager, Ryan Koski, who keeps me on the straight and narrow.

I count my blessings every day for my loving husband, Rick Lapine, who always sees the glass half full, and our beautiful children, Emily and Sam—you are my world.

Finally, to my Sneaky Chef community, I can't tell you how much I appreciate your trust in bringing my recipes and products into your home.

I am sincerely grateful to all of you.

Missy Chase Lapine

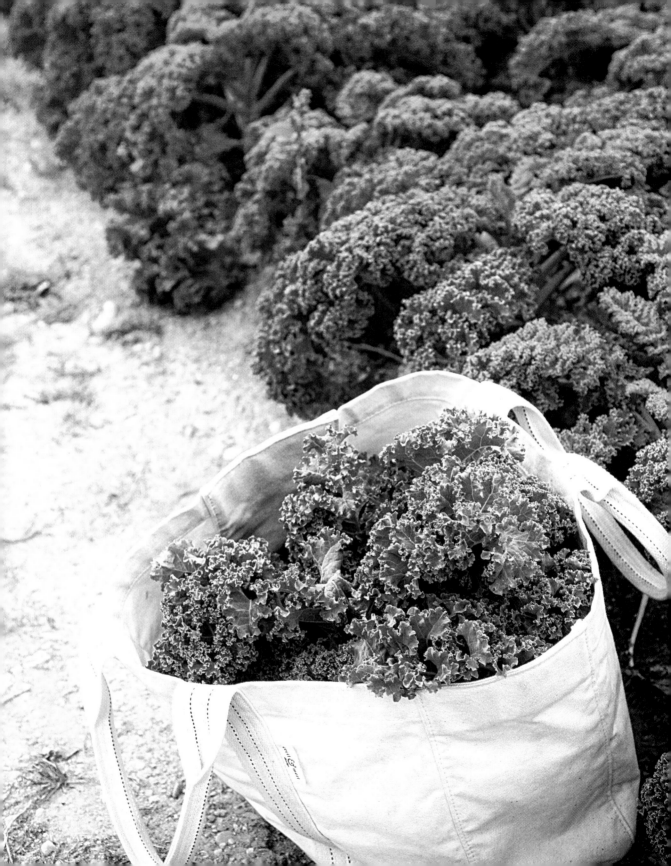

Conversion Chart

LIQUID MEASURES

Fluid Ounces	U.S.	Imperial	Milliliters
	1 teaspoon	1 teaspoon	5
¼	2 teaspoons	2 teaspoons	10
½	1 tablespoon	1 dessertspoon	14
1	2 tablespoons	2 tablespoons	28
2	¼ cup	4 tablespoons	56
4	½ cup		120
5		¼ pint or 1 gill	140
6	¾ cup		170
8	1 cup		240
9			250; ¼ liter
10	1 ¼ cups	½ pint	280
12	1 ½ cups		340
15		¾ pint	420
16	2 cups		450
18	2 ¼ cups		500; ½ liter
20	2 ½ cups	1 pint	560
24	3 cups		675
25		1 ¼ pints	700
27	3 ½ cups		750
30	3 ¾ cups	1 ½ pints	840
32	4 cups; 1 quart		900
35		1 ¾ pints	980
36	4 ½ cups		1000; 1 liter
40	5 cups	2 pints; 1 quart	1120

SOLID MEASURES

Ounces	Pounds	Grams	Kilos
1		28	
2		56	
3 ½		100	
4	¼	112	
5		140	
6		168	
8	½	225	
9		250	¼
12	¾	340	
16	1	450	
18		500	½
20	1 ¼	560	
24	1 ½	675	
27		750	¾
28	1 ¾	780	
32	2	900	
36	2 ¼	1000	1
40	2 ½	1100	
48	3	1350	
54		1500	1 ½

Recipe Index

Plate

Nibble

Sip

Indulge

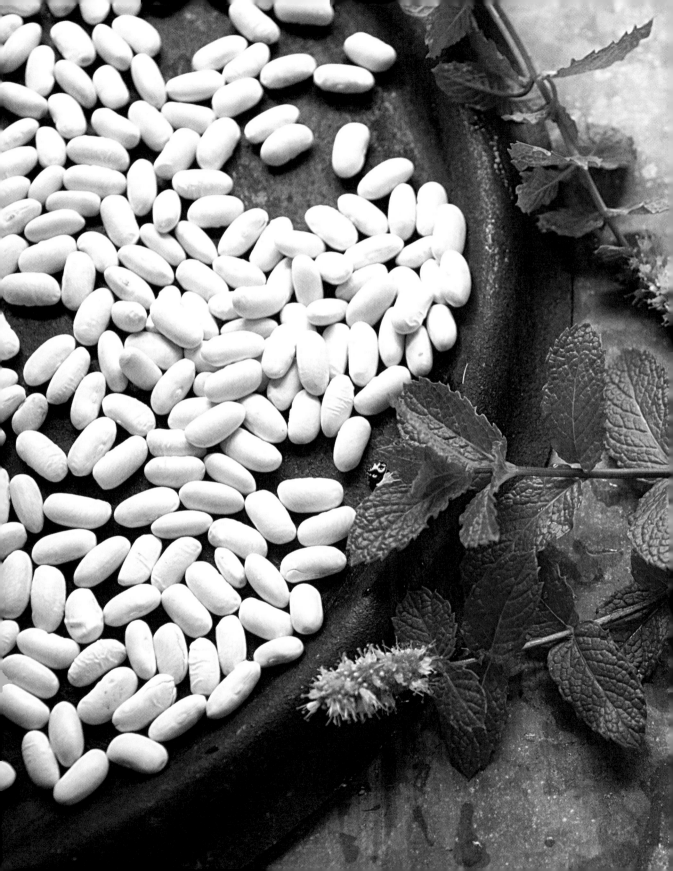

Recipe Index By Base Blend

Butternut Squash–Apple Base Blend

Carrot–Sweet Potato Base Blend

Cauliflower Base Blend

All Hail Eggless Caesar Dressing, 182
Artichoke–Kalamata Olive Hummus, 210
Bean and Goat Cheese Blend, 195
Cauliflower-Chive Blend, 196
Cauliflower-Chive Cleanse Blend, 46
Coconut Corn Chowder with Cilantro and Lime, 177
Crab and Artichoke Dip, 208
Creamy Feta Dressing, 185
Creamy Tomato-Basil Soup, 151
Crunchy Kale-Crust Pizza, 146
Kale Chips with Sour Cream and Onion Dip, 200
Roasted Red Pepper Hummus, 211
Zucchini Pasta Piccata, 158

Chickpea-Zucchini Base Blend

4 P.M. Protein Cookie, 207
All Hail Eggless Caesar Dressing, 182
Artichoke–Kalamata Olive Hummus, 210
Cauliflower Parmesan Biscuits, 199
Cinnamon-Oat Truffle Treats, 244
Citrus-Herb Roasted Turkey with Mushroom Gravy, 167
Cocoa-Cayenne Truffle Treats, 247
Coconut-Almond Truffle Treats, 246
Coconut Corn Chowder with Cilantro and Lime, 177
Crab and Artichoke Dip, 208
Creamy Tomato-Basil Soup, 151
Creamy White Bean "Butter" Dip, 216
Crunchy Kale-Crust Pizza, 146
Curried Chicken Salad–Stuffed Pitas, 178
Curried Deviled Eggs, 204
Miso-Kale Noodle Bowl, 175
"No More Muffin Top!" Blueberry Muffin Tops, 113
Parisian Tuna Salad, 149
Revamped Russian Dressing, 186
Roasted Red Pepper Hummus, 211
White Bean–Rosemary Cleanse Blend, 50
Zucchini Pasta Piccata, 158

Mixed Berry–Baby Kale Base Blend

5-a-Day Brownies, 243
Berry Detox Shake, 126
Chocolate Crepes, 109
Cocoa Protein Pancakes, 125
Coffee-Chia Brewsicles, 215
Creamy Berry Blend, 107
Mixed Berry–Kale Shake, 219
Mixed Berry Sorbet Blend, 229
Not Your Mom's (Turkey) Meat Loaf, 171
Purple Detox Lemonade, 221
Skinny Chocolate Cake, 249
Southwestern Turkey Burger, 145

Sweet Pea Base Blend

Broccoli-Cheddar Mini
    Frittata, 117
Cheesy Kale-Basil Soufflé,
    130
Creamy Kale Guac, 203
Even Greener Goddess
    Dressing, 183

Pesto Pasta with Roasted
    Shrimp, 168
Pistachio Power Pesto,
    190
Seared Salmon with Dill
    Sauce, 150

Spring Sweet Pea Soup,
    141
Thai-Style Blend, 139
Triple-Greens Cleanse
    Blend, 49
Warm Green Basil Blend,
    138

Sweet Pea–Baby Kale Base Blend

Broccoli-Cheddar Mini
    Frittata, 117
Cheesy Kale-Basil Soufflé,
    130
Creamy Kale Guac, 203

Even Greener Goddess
    Dressing, 183
Pesto Pasta With Roasted
    Shrimp, 168
Pistachio Power Pesto,
    190

Seared Salmon with Dill
    Sauce, 150
Thai-Style Blend, 139
Triple-Greens Cleanse
    Blend, 49
Warm Green Basil Blend,
    138

White Bean Base Blend

4 P.M. Protein Cookie,
    207
All Hail Eggless Caesar
    Dressing, 182
Artichoke–Kalamata
    Olive Hummus, 210
Bean and Goat Cheese
    Blend, 195
Cauliflower Parmesan
    Biscuits, 199
Cinnamon-Oat Truffle
    Treats, 244
Citrus-Herb Roasted
    Turkey with
    Mushroom Gravy, 167
Cocoa-Cayenne Truffle
    Treats, 247

Coconut-Almond Truffle
    Treats, 246
Coconut Corn Chowder
    with Cilantro and
    Lime, 177
Crab and Artichoke Dip,
    208
Creamy Tomato-Basil
    Soup, 151
Creamy White Bean
    "Butter" Dip, 216
Crunchy Kale-Crust
    Pizza, 146
Curried Chicken Salad–
    Stuffed Pitas, 178
Curried Deviled Eggs,
    204

Miso-Kale Noodle Bowl,
    175
"No More Muffin Top!"
    Blueberry Muffin
    Tops, 113
Parisian Tuna Salad, 149
Revamped Russian
    Dressing, 186
Roasted Red Pepper
    Hummus, 211
Rosemary–White Bean
    Blend, 195
White Bean–Rosemary
    Cleanse Blend, 50
Zucchini Pasta Piccata,
    158

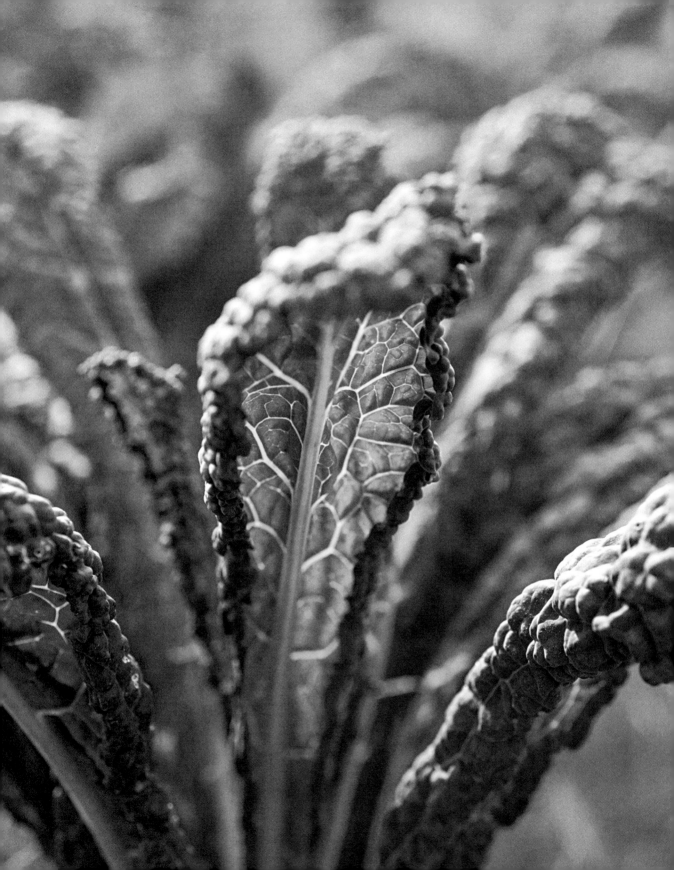

Index

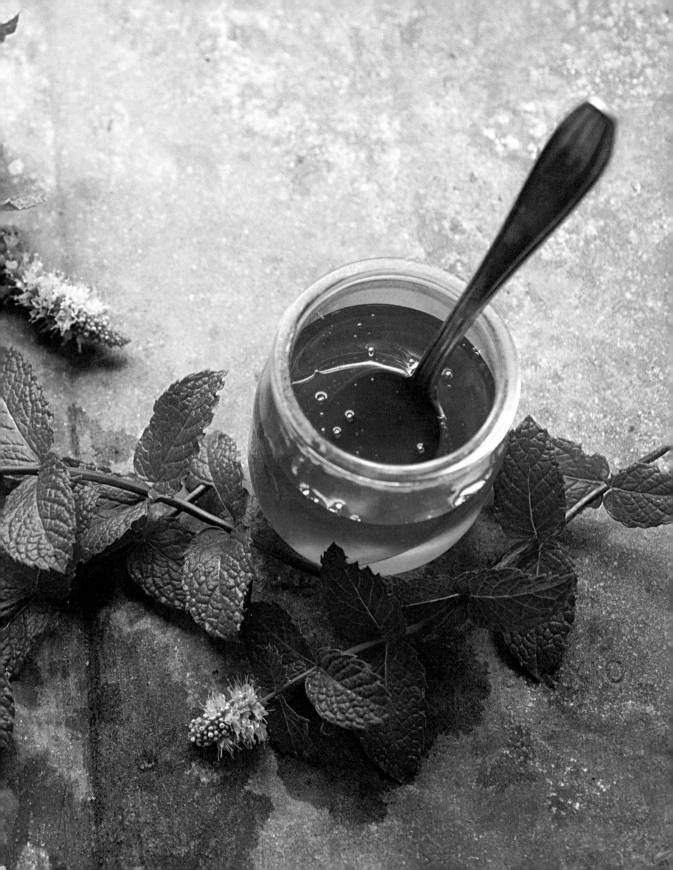

About the Author

Missy Chase Lapine is best known for her game-changing Sneaky Chef series of books, including her *New York Times* bestseller, *The Sneaky Chef: Simple Strategies for Hiding Healthy Foods in Kids' Favorite Meals*. Missy's fresh, proven approach has made The Sneaky Chef a household name with a passionate following—and has transformed the way America feeds its families.

In addition to her seven books, Missy is also the founder of Sneaky Chef Foods, LLC, a company committed to developing products that improve children's health by helping moms easily feed their kids the veggies they need in the foods they already love. Her products include Sneaky Chef No-Nut Butter and pasta sauces made with eight hidden veggies. Sneaky Chef foods are sold at various Target, Walmart, Albertsons, Stop & Shop, Publix, and natural grocers nationwide.

As a celebrity chef, Missy has appeared on *The Today Show* and has made hundreds of national TV, radio, and print appearances, and is a regular contributor to The Huffington Post and The Daily Meal. She is also a member of the Children's Advisory Council for NewYork-Presbyterian/Morgan Stanley Children's Hospital, where Sneaky Chef meals are served to patients. She lives in Westchester County, New York, with her husband and two daughters.

Missy's fresh, irreverent approach to nutrition comes through on her website, TheSneakyChef.com.